Program Evaluation

Program Evaluation

Forms and Approaches

Third Edition

JOHN M. OWEN

Foreword by Marvin C. Alkin

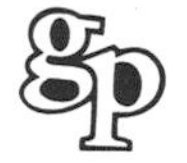

THE GUILFORD PRESS
New York London

Edition with Australian examples and spellings first published by
Allen & Unwin, Australia, 2006

Edition with U.S. examples and spellings published 2007 by
The Guilford Press
A Division of Guilford Publications, Inc.
72 Spring Street, New York, NY 10012
www.guilford.com

Printed in the United States of America

This book is printed on acid-free paper.

Last digit is print number: 9 8 7 6 5 4 3 2 1

Library of Congress Cataloging-in-Publication Data

Owen, John M.
Program evaluation : forms and approaches / John M. Owen. — 3rd ed.
p. cm.
Includes bibliographical references and index.
ISBN-13: 978-1-59385-411-9 (hardcover : alk. paper)
ISBN-10: 1-59385-411-0 (hardcover : alk. paper)
ISBN-13: 978-1-59385-406-5 (pbk. : alk. paper)
ISBN-10: 1-59385-406-4 (pbk. : alk. paper)
1. Project management—Evaluation. 2. Management—Evaluation. 3. Evaluation. 4. Evaluation—Methodology. I. Title.
HD69.P75O94 2007
658.4—dc22

2006024519

About the Author

John M. Owen, PhD, is Principal Fellow, Centre for Program Evaluation at the University of Melbourne, and was Director of the Centre from 1992 to 2002. He is a regular contributor to international journals and conferences and serves on the editorial boards of *Evaluation and Program Planning*, the *Evaluation Journal of Australasia*, and the *Canadian Journal of Program Evaluation*. In 2001, he was awarded a Universitas 21 Fellowship by the University of Melbourne for his work in developing an online graduate program in evaluation that attracts students from around the world. Dr. Owen has been a visiting scholar at the University of Oregon, the University of Maryland, and Hiroshima University. His interests in evaluation result from a long-standing concern for the effective application of social inquiry to organizational improvement and to policy and program delivery.

Contents

Foreword

Consider a patient under the care of a medical doctor. Assume that this 'health evaluator' adheres to a model of care that guides her every action—a specific evaluative protocol that she always follows . . . a rather silly assumption, but bear with me. During the initial visit, the patient complains of dizziness and mild chest pain. The doctor's main goal during this visit is to assess the symptoms and accurately diagnose the medical condition plaguing the patient. The doctor schedules a follow-up visit after the patient commences a prescribed drug therapy. The doctor's main goal for this visit is to ensure adherence to the treatment regimen and to examine early progress. During a final visit with the patient, the doctor is interested in determining whether the treatment therapy 'worked'. Clearly, each of the purposes of these visits, or 'health evaluations', is different. If, as stated in this hypothetical example, the doctor blindly followed the same model of care, or evaluation, for each interaction with our imaginary patient, she couldn't achieve her intended goals for each visit. Diagnosing an illness, monitoring a therapeutic intervention, and determining the effect all require different evaluative approaches and disparate data.

What this example brings to mind is how the particular purposes and aims of different evaluative situations intersect with the various evaluation theories currently prevalent in the field. Each evaluation starts with a specific goal, whether it is to diagnose, monitor, determine a treatment effect, or any other of the numerous possibilities. Additionally, each evaluator approaches an evaluation with a particular philosophical perspective about the nature of evaluation. I refer to these perspectives on evaluation as 'theories' in my book *Evaluation Roots* (Alkin 2004). In fact, they are prescriptive theories. That is, there are evaluation luminaries who have prescribed what they believe to be the proper way to conduct an evaluation based on the assumptions they make about the role of evaluation and aspects that they deem to be important. Good evaluators, however, don't let their perspectives or models blind them like our hypothetical Dr. One-Size-Fits-All health evaluator. Rather, good evaluators use their philosophical perspectives as a guide to be adapted depending on the goals, aims, and contexts of each evaluative situation.

John Owen was confronted with the 'one-size-fits-all' issue some years ago when he began teaching a new graduate program in evaluation to individuals experienced in middle management, and with a new responsibility for evaluation in their organizations but without any prior training in evaluation. As the students were introduced to evaluation models and approaches, they found that the material wasn't necessarily relevant to the particular circumstances they faced. The question became: Should an evaluator adhere to a specific evaluation approach for all situations? Owen noticed that 'neophyte evaluators . . . had great difficulty in marrying those models to the practical needs of their work places' (2004, p. 361). He was concerned that new practitioners 'would latch on to one of these models no matter what the circumstances, and regardless of the lack of congruence between the model proposed and the knowledge needs of stakeholder' (2004, p. 361). While it should be noted that some evaluation models can be adapted to different circumstances and situations, it is difficult for a novice to recognize the need to do so or how to make the modifications. What is a better way to guide the actions of novice evaluators?

In addressing this issue, Owen maintains that it is important to understand the 'what' and the 'why' of an evaluation and select the distinct 'epistemological cluster' that best fits the issues that need to be addressed in the evaluation. He refers to these clusters as 'Forms'. Unlike the stages of evaluation depicted by Daniel Stufflebeam in his CIPP model, the Forms are not necessarily sequential but rather *situational*, and provide the basis for structuring activities. The metamodel that Owen created, and which is the basis for this book, consists of five Forms: (1) Proactive (e.g. needs assessment, best practices), (2) Clarificative (e.g. logic development), (3) Interactive (e.g. particular involvement in examining adequacy of implementation), (4) Monitoring (e.g. documenting the program in operation), and (5) Impact (e.g. effects of a program). Each of these Forms has relevant methods and key approaches associated with it. Each Form has a different epistemological basis consisting of different purposes, assumptions, and imperatives. For example, a Form called 'Monitoring' has the purpose of checking/refining/accountability. The assumption within this Form is that programs need to be monitored to ensure quality, leading to the imperative of the importance of quality control.

In Owen's presentation of evaluation practice, programs are presented not as static entities on which to blindly apply standard social science methods or a single evaluation perspective, but rather as dynamic entities with different needs at different times. Owen insightfully captures these complexities of evaluative work and outlines, in an accessible format, all the many considerations needed in order to truly serve the information needs of all sorts of evaluands. Perhaps most important, Owen begins his work with a helpful synthesis of the general logic of evaluation both implicit and explicit. This overview benefits even the most experienced evaluators.

Owen rightly contrasts evaluation with research. He points out that evaluation requires the necessity of involving stakeholders in the planning process. In one of the best chapters in the book, Owen goes beyond the notion of stakeholder involvement to examine, in depth, the nature of and skills required in negotiating with stakeholders. Most specifically, he considers skills related to negotiating the evaluation plan. All client questions cannot be answered by an evaluation and choices must be made. Moreover, a concerned evaluator pays heed to how the evaluation might ultimately be used. This too is a topic for negotiation. Managers of any evaluation will appreciate his practical and detailed advice about negotiating with clients at the beginning stages of an evaluation.

Owen successfully achieves his goal of making this guide very practical by including a variety of examples and closely integrating evaluation with the management perspectives and functions. These examples are from a great variety of contexts—subject fields, program types, and geographic locations—providing a very broad perspective on evaluation. Furthermore, examples are elaborated to reinforce the discussion in the text. In some instances, mini-scenarios are constructed that demand attention and force readers to think actively.

In creating a volume that outlines the logic of evaluation and the many considerations that influence an evaluation effort, and then subsequently details the many practical aspects of evaluation work, Owen provides practitioners with the tools that ultimately empower them to take leadership roles in evaluation projects. This move from passive recipient to empowered leader is particularly critical in the current climate of accountability. As programs are expected to 'prove' their worth, it is a noble mission to arm program staff with sophisticated understandings of evaluation practice. In doing so, Owen's work strives to better the field of evaluation as a whole by raising practitioners' expectations of evaluators. Reading Owen's presentation of evaluation practice gives one a deep sense of the innate possibility of evaluation in the service of program improvement. The spirit of this work captures at the most fundamental level why most of us do this work.

MARVIN C. ALKIN, EdD
Professor Emeritus, University of California, Los Angeles

REFERENCES

Alkin, M. C. (ed) (2004). *Evaluation Roots: Tracing Theorists' Views and Influences*. Thousand Oaks, CA: Sage.

Owen, J. M. (2004). Evaluation Forms: Toward an Inclusive Framework for Evaluation Practice. In M.C. Alkin (ed), *Evaluation Roots: Tracing Theorists' Views and Influences* (pp. 356-369). Thousand Oaks, CA: Sage.

Preface

About 15 years ago, I began teaching in a graduate program in evaluation. The program was a response to a need for knowledge and skills in evaluation by those wanting to commission or undertake evaluations in organizational settings. The typical student entering this program already had an undergraduate degree and some years of experience in middle management, and had been given responsibility for job-related evaluation tasks. While these students had limited knowledge of evaluation theory, the evaluation work experiences that students brought to class were many and varied.

Working with these students, I began to find that their needs could not be always be satisfied by my existing expertise, which was based on the assumption that evaluation was only about assessing the worth of mature programs. The students were thinking about and undertaking evaluations in real life. Often, a decision needed to be made under pressure of time. Associated with time-related decisions, many interventions, policies, programs, and services were not mature or established. These evaluations reflected the need for information that could be used directly to influence the structure of an intervention and its implementation.

About this time, I attended a conference of the American Evaluation Society and heard Michael Scriven make a distinction between evaluation, as the determination of worth, and 'what evaluators do'. There were many other evaluators who were and still are writing about what evaluators do, but no one had tried to tie all these contributions together. This book attempts to do this in two ways.

The first is to present a metamodel of evaluation by providing a conceptual map for the full range of practical applications of evaluation in contemporary settings. This epistemological map comprises Evaluation Forms, a heuristic that reduces the complexity facing evaluators and program stakeholders when they plan and implement an evaluation study. An important implication is that evaluation findings have a range of orientations or applications vis-à-vis the program under review. Each Form represents a type of knowledge production activity consistent with this orientation. The Forms provide a 'first-order' conceptual comparison of the range of contemporary evaluation practice—a between-Forms analysis, if you like. Also, each Form provides an umbrella for a cluster of several theoretical models or approaches that also have a common orientation. This encourages an invitation to explore theoretical differences within each Form, should the reader wish to do so by following the references provided at the end of each chapter.

While this first contribution is about knowledge production, the second is about nesting knowledge production within a framework of intentionality. I argue that attention to stakeholder/evaluator negotiation and to dissemination are integral aspects of effective evaluation practice. An important implication is that evaluators must come to possess important interpersonal and communication skills, in addition to developing a repertoire of social inquiry skills, in order to be effective. These are elements that have received scant attention in many previous evaluation texts, and are rarely covered in graduate programs that purport to prepare practicing evaluators. This book extends ideas about negotiation over and above those put forward by fourth-generation theorists and provides an integrated model of utilization that summarizes and builds on the extensive previous treatment of the topic.

ORGANIZATION OF THE BOOK

The book consists of 13 chapters. Chapters 1 and 4–8 provide an overview of issues common to all evaluation studies. Chapter 1 develops an argument for a contemporary definition of evaluation that involves key elements: negotiation, evaluation design, and dissemination. Chapters 4–6 are devoted to an extensive discussion of each of these elements in turn. Chapters 7 and 8 provide information about managing evaluations and dealing with the ethical and political aspects of evaluation practice. In keeping with the intention of the book to link evaluation with effective interventions, Chapter 2 examines and compares the nature of intervention: policies, programs, and products. Chapter 3 uses a framework for introducing the Forms and discusses each of them in turn. Key models or approaches within each Form are introduced. Chapters 9–13 are devoted to theory and practice related to one Form, referenced to the appropriate ideas developed in Chapters 1–8. They also include a section on trends and case studies to link practice with theory.

Notwithstanding this logic, most chapters can be read independently of others, so that the book can be used as a source or reference for program managers and evaluators wishing to access a specific topic of interest.

NEW OR REVISED TOPICS

This book is based on a previous edition that was published in 1999. While the structure of this edition is basically the same, modifications have been made to reflect changes in the evaluation knowledge base. Chapter 7 has been included in response to the need for information about evaluation management. Within each chapter, new sections have been added to reflect the increased interest in topics such as negotiation theory, evidence-based practice, performance auditing and management, and realistic evaluation.

AUDIENCE

This book is designed for a first course in a graduate program in evaluation and as a resource for students undertaking master's and doctoral theses. The previous edition has also been used as the text in professional development courses for practitioners and as a sourcebook for program managers, practicing evaluators, and performance auditors.

PEDAGOGICAL FEATURES

The book is designed to be reader friendly, using a conversational style consistent with what is known about good practice in adult education. Each chapter contains boxed examples to illustrate key points of theory and a list of references that enable the student or practitioner to access the work of other theorists in the area covered by that chapter.

It is important to note that this is not a book about methodology or methods. Most of the examples, however, incorporate references to data collection and analysis techniques. This is designed to emphasize that while social inquiry is an important aspect, evaluation practice should be issues driven rather than methodologically driven.

Acknowledgments

This book would not be possible without the environment of ideas and practice of staff at the Centre for Program Evaluation at the University of Melbourne. A special note of thanks to the following colleagues and friends: Pamela Andrew, Rosalind Hurworth, Neil Day, Pam St Leger, Bradley Shrimpton, John McLeod, Ian Ling, Carole Hooper, Marion Brown, Tanner LeBaron Wallace, and Marvin C. Alkin. I would also like to acknowledge C. Deborah Laughton at The Guilford Press for her advice and persistence in making this version of the book come to fruition. Finally, I would like to recognize my colleagues from the international evaluation community for their constructive feedback about the ideas presented in previous versions of this book.

Figures and Tables

FIGURES

TABLES

1 Evaluation Fundamentals

This book is based on the premise that evaluation, as defined in this and following chapters, can and should enhance the quality of interventions (policies and programs) designed to solve or ameliorate problems in social and corporate settings. Evaluation should be seen as a process of knowledge production, which rests on the use of rigorous empirical inquiry. Evaluation will be worth the investment of time and money if the knowledge produced is reliable, responsive to the needs of policy and program stakeholders, and can be applied by these stakeholders.

Evaluation is not an alien activity for most of us. We engage informally in evaluative activity in our everyday lives. What clothes to wear on a given day, whether the plans for home renovations are satisfactory, how the new worker in the office is coping, whether our sporting team played well, are all examples of evaluation in our daily lives. In most of these examples, the evaluation is performed informally, for private purposes. That is, we often assemble information 'in our heads' based on a variety of sensory inputs, such as observation, and our existing knowledge, to make judgments about the issue under consideration. For example, an evaluation of how the new worker in the office is coping may rely on informal observations of performance and the opinions of others, including the worker herself.

This book should assist you to extrapolate your everyday understandings to more formal evaluation frameworks and procedures than those just mentioned. A comprehensive conceptual framework for anchoring your existing evaluation knowledge and practice is put forward. We have adopted an eclectic view of the field in order that you:

- may also see new directions for evaluation work; and can
- identify aspects of evaluation theory and practice that you wish to

explore in more detail. This can be achieved by following up the relevant concepts and ideas through the references provided at the end of each chapter.

There is no doubt that evaluation practice has expanded and become more complex during the period of more than fifty years since the first formal evaluations were undertaken. Our intention is to encapsulate this complexity into a format that is both understandable and workable for you.

THE LOGIC OF EVALUATION

At the outset, we introduce you to what has been termed the 'logic of evaluation'. Anyone interested in undertaking or commissioning evaluative work must be familiar with this logic. We can anchor the logic of evaluation in the everyday scheme of things by asking you to read the following extract from a 'test report' on breakfast cereals, typical of those found in *Consumer Reports* in the United States. The intervention or 'object' being evaluated here is a product, something that we buy to use or consume. Specifically, the extract describes the evaluation of a range of breakfast cereals.

When reading this extract, think about the following issues:

- What is the underlying basis for selecting criteria to judge the worth of each breakfast cereal?
- What evidence was used and on what standards was the judgment of worth made?
- How were the conclusions made and presented?
- Decision-making: you have been asked to recommend one brand of cereal to members of your household or to a friend. Which one will you choose?

Example 1.1 Test report: Evaluating breakfast cereals

Most of us eat them, but just how healthy are they? We've assessed more than 80 breakfast cereals to find out which are the most nutritious, and compared them to other breakfast options.

Breakfast is probably the most important meal of the day, but it's generally the most neglected one. By morning, around ten hours have usually passed since you last ate, so your body is running low on fuel. You need to replenish your stores, or your performance will suffer.

Studies have shown that by lunchtime, people who eat breakfast are functioning better than those who don't. Adults who haven't eaten breakfast are more likely to be involved in industrial accidents, and children who miss this meal suffer significant drops in concentration levels in the late morning.

Breakfast-eaters are also more likely to eat well throughout the rest of the day than those who give it a miss. If you meet your nutritional needs at the start of the day, you're less likely to binge on sweet or fatty snacks later in the day. If you're trying to lose weight, there's another reason you shouldn't miss breakfast: studies have shown when you do, the body's metabolic rate remains lower for the rest of the day—and with a low metabolic rate you burn fuel more slowly so you're not shedding those pounds.

The ideal breakfast

It's also important to feed your body the right kind of fuel in the morning. The best breakfast is one that is high in complex carbohydrate. Once digested, carbohydrate is stored in the muscles and liver as glycogen, a convenient storage form of glucose, which your body can then draw on throughout the day to fuel mental and physical activity.

Unprocessed cereals and grains—the starting point of breakfast cereals—fit this bill perfectly. They are high in complex carbohydrate, as well as being a good source of protein, fiber, vitamins and minerals.

But how nutritious are they after they've been processed, when things are often added to them or taken away? We looked at more than 80 breakfast cereals, assessing their nutritional profiles to find which are the most and the least nutritious.

There are thousands of different breakfast cereal products on the market, so we weren't able to look at them all. Our selection includes those widely available in supermarkets and all the top sellers in the ready-to-eat segment.

What makes a good breakfast cereal?

A nutritious breakfast cereal should be low in fat, sugar and salt as well as high in complex carbohydrate and dietary fiber. Some of the processed cereals on the market have retained many of the nutritional virtues of the original whole grain. But many more have had fat, sugar and salt added to them. Some have also had other nutrients added to them, often ones which were naturally in the original grain but were lost during processing, like fiber and thiamine (vitamin B1).

All up, we found 30 cereals that are a good choice to eat for breakfast; the data on these cereals are included in Table 1.1.

Figures given are those supplied by manufacturers in their nutrition panels, except for the fiber content of Kellogg's Puffed Wheat which was determined by laboratory analysis. Numbers were rounded to the nearest whole number in order to place products into ranking categories, e.g., 19.3 percent was considered to be 19 percent.

How the cereals were rated

Ideally, we would want a branded breakfast cereal to provide similar levels of nutrients to uncooked wholegrain cereals. We looked at the nutrient profiles of some of these raw cereals and used them as a starting point for developing a model for ranking the breakfast cereals. For details of the amounts of each nutrient in our 'highly recommended', 'recommended', 'OK' and 'not recommended' cereals, see below. A product had to meet our requirements for all four nutrients—fat, sugar, fiber and sodium—to get into a category, not just for one of them.

1 *Fiber* Fiber is an important part of the diet: it adds bulk, which helps you to feel full and satisfied, and helps with the elimination of wastes from the body. Too little fiber in the diet leads to constipation, and has also been suggested as a contributory factor in some cancers, particularly of the breast and colon. To be highly recommended or recommended, a cereal had to contain 7 percent or more fiber. To be OK it had to have a least 3 percent fiber; anything less than this meant the cereal was not recommended.
2 *Fat* To be rated as highly recommended, a cereal had to contain 4 percent or less fat; to be recommended or OK it had to have 9 percent or less. Packaged cereals which are more than 9 percent fat were not recommended. Fat should be kept to a minimum in the diet. It's the most energy-dense nutrient, and excessive consumption is linked to diet-related conditions like obesity, heart disease, diabetes and some cancers. Generally, it's recommended that fat should contribute no more than 30 percent of your total energy intake. However, infants, preschool children, underweight people, lactating women and those who do unusually heavy work may need more than this.

3 *Sugars* Unprocessed cereals have a naturally low sugar content—we considered less than the 5 percent the maximum for highly recommended products. This figure also takes into account the increase in sugar content that would occur through loss of moisture when the cereals are processed (which makes the nutrients more concentrated). For a cereal to be rated as recommended or OK, the amount of sugar had to be 19 percent or less. This represents the 5 percent plus the equivalent of an extra teaspoon per serve. Anything over 19 percent and the cereal fell into the not recommended category. If you sprinkle much more than a teaspoon of sugar onto your bowl of some of these cereals, you could turn them into the equivalent of not recommended.
4 *Sodium* Sodium may be found in some breakfast cereals in the form of common salt (sodium chloride), sodium bicarbonate or other compounds. Current knowledge suggests a high sodium intake is linked with the development of high blood pressure, stroke and coronary heart disease in susceptible people. Recent overseas studies have shown that salt added by food manufacturers makes up the bulk of most people's daily intake, so it is important to watch out for high-sodium cereals, particularly if you eat a lot of other processed foods.

Just how much salt is too much is not clear. The amount we chose for a cereal to be recommended or OK—600 mg or less of sodium per 100 g—is not overly strict. If a cereal contained 600 mg per 100 g, a 30 g serve would contribute one-fifth of the lower recommended dietary intake (RDI) of sodium. (The RDI for sodium is expressed as a range; we used the amount at the lower end of the range as our guide.)

Findings

Many cereals have a very short list of ingredients, indicating they are fairly close to their original, unprocessed counterparts in terms of nutritional characteristics. We split the 30 into 'highly recommended' and 'recommended' categories: the difference between these two groups was that, to be highly recommended, a cereal had to contain less fat and sugar. Overall, we based our evaluation on the amount of fiber the cereals contain (the more the better), and the amount of fat, sugar and salt (the less the better):

- *Fiber*: All the top 30 were a good source; the two that fell into the OK category in our table contained less but were still a reasonable source.

Table 1.1 Characteristics of breakfast cereals

Brand/type (alphabetically within groups)	Category	Fiber (g/) all = per 100g	Fat (g/)	Sugars (g/)	Sodium (mg/)	Carbo (g/)	Energy (kj/cal/)
Highly recommended (4% or less fat, 5% or less sugar, 7% or more fiber, 600 mg/100 g or less sodium)							
HOME BRAND Wheat Biscuits	Biscuit	12.2	2.7	2.3	270.0	64.5	1380/330
KELLOGG'S Mini-Wheats Whole Wheat	Shredded wheat	9.3	2.6	0.9	3.0	77.1	1523/363
KELLOGG'S Wholegrain Wheat Flakes	Wheat-based	11.0	1.1	2.0	468.0	81.3	1437/382
SANITARIUM Lite-bix	'Light'	12.0	2.7	1.2	20.0	62.0	1340/320
SANITARIUM Puffed Wheat	Wheat-based	7.5	2.6	1.0	17.0	71.0	1440/344
SANITARIUM Weet-Bix	Biscuit	12.2	2.7	2.3	270.0	64.5	1380/330
UNCLE TOBYS Organic Vita-Brits	Biscuit	12.4	1.4	1.8	400.0	65.6	1320/315
UNCLE TOBYS Shredded Wheat	Shredded wheat	13.2	1.2	2.0	8.0	82.0	1330/318
UNCLE TOBYS Wheeties	Wheat-based	10.1	1.4	2.5	340.0	69.8	1390/332
Recommended (9% or less fat, 19% or less sugar, 7% or more fiber, 600 mg/100 g or less sodium)							
GOODNESS Tropical Toasted Muesli	Toasted muesli	7.4	8.7	15.4	9.0	51.5	1569/375
KELLOGG'S Just Right	Combination	9.3	1.4	18.2	295.0	65.0	1534/381
KELLOGG'S Mini-Wheats Apricot	Shredded wheat	11.9	1.1	16.4	26.0	66.5	1503/358
KELLOGG'S Sustain	Sports	7.5	2.9	15.0	112.0	67.8	1607/399
LOWAN Australian Rolled Oats (A)	Rolled oats	11.5	8.7	1.2	6.3	65.3	1624/388
MORNING SUN Natural Apricot and Almond Muesli	Natural muesli	17.6	8.3	17.8	32.0	51.4	1420/339
THE OLD GRAIN MILL Australian Gold Classic Muesli	Natural muesli	12.2	8.7	19.3	46.0	46.7	1610/385

Brand/type (alphabetically within groups)	Category	Fiber (g/) all = per 100g	Fat (g/)	Sugars (g/)	Sodium (mg/)	Carbo (g/)	Energy (kj/cal/)
THE OLD GRAIN MILL Australian Gold Natural Muesli	Natural muesli	11.9	6.3	17.5	66.0	56.5	1548/370
SANITARIUM Bran Bix	Biscuit	22.0	4.4	5.7	410.0	45.0	1180/280
SANITARIUM Crunchy Bix	Biscuit	7.7	5.5	13.0	320.0	58.7	16/380
SANITARIUM Natural Muesli	Natural muesli	7.1	5.1	18.6	124.0	44.0	1400/333
SANITARIUM Weet-Bix plus Oat Bran	Biscuit	11.6	4.8	7.3	250.0	54.7	1440/345
UNCLE TOBYS Crunchy Oat Bran	Bran	15.0	5.8	16.6	240.0	51.2	1499/358
UNCLE TOBYS Hi-Fiber Oats	Rolled oats	12.9	9.0	<1.0	5.0	58.3	1500/358
UNCLE TOBYS Instant Porridge (A)	Rolled oats	10.0	9.2	0.5	<5.0	61.3	1530/366
UNCLE TOBYS Muesli Flakes	Combination	9.0	2.6	19.0	240.0	53.9	1390/332
UNCLE TOBYS Natural Apricot & Almond Muesli	Natural muesli	13.8	8.3	17.8	30.0	41.4	1420/339
WEIGHT WATCHERS Fruit & Fiber Cereal	'Light'	11.8	2.5	18.5	170.0	60.0	1495/357
WILLOW VALLEY Multi Bran	Bran	36.3	9.3	12.8	122.0	57.4	1727/413
OK (9% or less fat, 19% or less sugar, 3% to 6.5% fiber, 600 mg/100 g or less sodium)							
KELLOGG'S Puffed Wheat	Wheat-based	6.0	2.3	1.1	3.0	78.1	1614/385
KELLOGG'S Special K	'Light'	2.9	0.5	14.4	475.0	57.7	1436/379

Source: Reprinted from CHOICE, January 1994 with the permission of the Australian Consumers' Association (ACA).

- *Fat*: Oats naturally contain more fat than other 'raw' cereals; although the fat levels of oat-based cereals kept them out of our highly recommended category, they're still a good choice for breakfast.
- *Sugar*: Our nine highly recommended cereals had little or no added sugar. Some people might put more on them, but we rated them without extra sugar. Most of the others in the table contain more sugar than these nine—around a teaspoon more per serving than naturally occurs in whole grains. For some brands it was contributed by dried fruit, which has a health advantage over cane sugar as it contributes some extra fiber.
- *Sodium*: The top 30 contained only small amounts of sodium. Common salt is sodium chloride and it's the sodium that's considered the problem.

Review

Let us go back to our questions, and your answers, with a view to 'pulling apart' the evaluation exercise (Example 1.1). Later we will review this exercise using some concepts developed by evaluation theorists.

- What is the underlying basis for selecting criteria to judge the worth of each cereal?

It is clear that the evaluators set up their criteria assuming that a nutritious breakfast is a 'good' breakfast. They believe that such a breakfast is important to give you a 'good start' and to sustain you throughout the day. Additionally, they claim that a nutritious breakfast is also one that will help you stay away from snacks that encourage you to put on weight. In a nutshell, the evaluators placed a high value on nutrition when setting up their criteria.

- What evidence was used and on what standards was the judgment of worth made?

The value position of the evaluator was translated into the selection of four characteristics for each cereal: fiber, fat, sugar and sodium. Variables or indicators were created for each characteristic, and data were collected on each indicator. In addition, data on complex carbohydrate and energy provision were also collected. The evaluator was able to access these data from the information provided on the packets of the cereals. Note that a cereal was more likely to be recommended if it was higher on fiber and lower on the other three variables.

Acceptable levels needed to classify a given cereal as 'good' were derived from the nutrient profiles of uncooked (raw) cereals. Note that, for each of the four variables, this *external* frame of reference provides the criterion for ranking the cereals and ultimately placing them in categories.

- How were the conclusions made and presented?

For each of these variables, those cereals that met standards on all four variables were ranked and classified as highly recommended, recommended, or OK. Note that the evidence for each of the four key variables was displayed along with the additional data on complex carbohydrates and energy provision.

- Decision-making: you have been asked to recommend one brand of cereal (to your household or a friend). Which one will you choose?

The evaluator has gone as far as categorizing the cereals and pointing out nine that are recommended. But for this last aspect of our case study, it is now over to you—or, in context, the readers of the article. Ultimately the choice of which cereal to buy will depend on the decision-making of the reader. Choosing one cereal from those highly recommended may depend on which of the criteria is more important to the reader—for example, there may be a preference for the cereal with the lowest sodium level, independent of the levels of the other variables. It could also be that a reader may choose on the basis of energy provision, that is, selecting the cereal within the highly recommended group that is highest on this variable.

EXTRAPOLATING TO A PROGRAM EVALUATION

The discussion above provides us with a basis for understanding the *logic of evaluation*. This is a logic that is consistent with a description of evaluation as the process of making a judgment about the value or worth of an object under review. At this stage it is worth noting that evaluators use the term 'evaluand' to generically denote the 'object' that is the focus for the evaluation.

Fournier (1995) summarized what we have done above very nicely when she describes the logic of evaluation as follows:

- *Establishing criteria of worth*
  - On what dimensions must the evaluand do well?
- *Constructing standards*
  - How well should the evaluand perform?

- *Measuring performance and comparing with standards*
  - How well did the evaluand perform?
- *Synthesizing and integrating evidence into a judgment of merit or worth*
  - What is the worth of the evaluand? (p. 16)

Fournier argues that this logic is appealing because of its generality. However what counts as criteria, how standards are set, what evidence is invoked, and how information is synthesized will, of course, vary for each evaluand. Fournier also notes that the logic can be applied within different fields, by which she means product evaluation, program evaluation, policy evaluation and personnel evaluation, which we would prefer to label as 'assessment' or 'appraisal'. The generality of the logic is its strength, for it gives us a base from which we can delve into different approaches to evaluation practice.

While the logic of evaluation might seem to simplify the work of an evaluator, the reality is that in practical evaluations, the evaluator must make a series of interrelated decisions in order to make a judgment of worth. Take the cereals case study above. In setting up the criteria the evaluators made it clear that the position adopted was that breakfasts should be nutritious. In good evaluations, value positions which frame the remainder of the evaluation should be made explicit, but in practice this is rarely the case (Kirkhart & Ruffolo 1993). Making the value base explicit is important because the conclusions follow from the value position taken, and those for whom the evaluation is intended must be aware of the value system that has undergirded the evaluation.

For example, if we had wanted to rank cereals that young children *preferred* to eat for breakfast, this would have had implications for the remainder of the evaluative process—the collection and analysis of data and the judgments that followed. You could imagine that the data collection would not be built around determining fiber and salt content. Rather, a key variable would be the satisfaction that children reported from eating different cereals! The standard might be a point on the upper end of a 'delicious' scale. The recommendation list would almost certainly have been different.

We should comment at this point about making a judgment of worth. Scriven (1971) insists that it behooves us to make a 'simple' judgment about an evaluand:

> It's [the evaluator's] task to try very hard to condense all that mass of data into one word: good or bad. Sometimes this is really impossible, but all too often the failure to do so is simply a cop-out disguised as or rationalized as objectivity (p. 53).

Figure 1.1 Conference evaluation: excerpt from questionnaire

Session 2: Science & Technology Policy Directions and Initiatives

Thinking about this session, to what extent:

- has your knowledge of the rationale and operation of this policy/initiative increased as a result of attending this workshop?

  not at all | a little | some | a lot | a great deal

- has your understanding of how the policy/initiative fits into the overall scheme of science/technology education in the state increased?

  not at all | a little | some | a lot | a great deal

- were the underlying professional development principles made clear in the presentation of the policy/initiative?

  not at all | a little | some | a lot | a great deal

- could you (or were you able to) explain the major features of the policy/initiative to a consultant who did not attend the session?

  not at all | a little | some | reasonably | comprehensively

- are you confident of being able to follow up on the policy/initiative if the need arises in your work?

  not at all | a little | somewhat | a lot | a great deal

- Do you have additional questions about the policy/initiative which need to be answered before you could use the information in your work? If so, jot them down below.

  ____

  ____

  ____

In our example, the evaluator has used a 'recommendation scale' and placed each of the cereals along this scale to indicate worth. This is really a refinement of Scriven's position, and paves the way for the evaluation audience to exercise some discretion in making a decision on the basis of the findings. Also, while the logic of evaluation is based on making judgments of worth about one evaluand, this evaluation provides findings about many evaluands.

In practice, criteria for judging the worth of a program could be drawn from:

- the program objectives;
- the needs of program clients, those for whom the program is intended;
- the objectives of a policy within which the program is nested;

Table 1.2 Conference evaluation: comparative impact of sessions 1–4

	1	2	3	4
	Trends in Professional Development	Science/ Technology Policy Directions	Math/ Technology Policy Directions	Regional Responses to SM&T
Knowledge of the rationale and operation of projects within theme	58	61	63	80
Understanding of how policy/initiative fits into overall state scheme	–	39	51	–
Clarity of underlying professional development principles	79	36	51	68
Ability to explain the major features to a colleague	91	72	64	86
Willing/confident to follow up on the project	68	49	58	71

Note: Each figure in the table is the percentage of participants responding to the item on the highest two points of a five-point scale (generally 'a lot' and 'a great deal').

- the preferences of one or more stakeholder groups; or
- efficiency measures, such as return on investment.

In summary, the notion of values as the basis for the practice of evaluation based on this logic cannot be overstated. The issue which then arises is: Whose values or value frame will be used to make judgments about a given evaluand? You can see that the selection of this frame is vital. When different value positions are held among the stakeholders (those who have an interest in the evaluand), a great deal can hang on the choice of the value perspective chosen. This has implications for practice and represents a challenge for evaluators to handle this diversity of views when negotiating and planning the evaluation (see Chapter 4).

EXPLICIT OR IMPLICIT LOGIC

Setting standards or levels of performance that an evaluand must attain to be judged as worthy is also fundamental to the evaluation logic. Ideally, these levels should be made explicit—in the evaluation in Example 1.1, they were set by referring to nationally accepted levels of nutrition for unprocessed cereals.

Owen and Downtown (1990) evaluated a large-scale training conference for educational consultants that was designed to provide them with information to use in their day-to-day work in schools. Conference organizers wished to gauge participant reactions to all seven major sessions of the conference and to the quality of the conference overall.

The major form of data collection was a structured questionnaire. All participants were given time at the end of the conference to complete it, after the evaluators had emphasized the importance of the feedback data. A page of the questionnaire is included as Figure 1.1.

Data were coded, analyzed and presented in tables as part of a written report. The findings for sessions 1–4 of the conference are reproduced as Table 1.2.

The four criteria presented (compare this with Example 1.1) were important from the point of view of the conference organizers in judging the worth of the conference. We chose to present findings on these criteria as the percentage of respondents who responded on the highest two points on the five-point scale.

To establish the effectiveness of each session we inspected the findings, as set out on Table 1.2, in conjunction with the conference organizers. It was clear that the organizers looked for patterns of responses for particular sessions and, as could be expected, they regarded session 1 as the 'most successful'. All analyses were comparative; there was little discussion as to whether any individual session was successful in its own right. This was almost certainly due to the fact that neither the evaluators nor the organizers considered, in advance of the data collection, the level of response needed for an individual session to be judged as successful—that is, standards were *not set explicitly.* One plausible standard was that, unless two-thirds of respondents (66 percent) responded favorably on all criteria, a session would not be regarded as 'worthy'. Using this standard, none of the sessions would be regarded as worthy and the conference would logically be regarded as a failure. Note, however, that if those judging the sessions chose to accept this standard as applied to the fifth criterion only, two of the sessions would be regarded as successful. This highlights the interaction between criteria and standards. In summary, there are no absolute criteria or standards, they need to be derived from some source. For example, one source of criteria is the objectives of an evaluand.

When the findings were actually presented, the organizers decided that the conference as a whole had gone well. We surmise that the conference organizers came to accept a standard which was less demanding than the one we have just mentioned, and furthermore that the standard, far from being set out formally, was implicit and shared by those concerned. In practice, many evaluations actually operate on a more informal interpretation of the logic of evaluation, a finding reported elsewhere (Fournier 1995).

The application of the logic of evaluation to real settings involves the evaluator, client or some other stakeholder holding a view about the worth of a given program based on defensible empirical inquiry. However, as a program needs to have been implemented, or 'in place', for such a judgment to be made, evaluations which are based on the logic of evaluation must lag behind program development, and are thus retrospective in nature. The logic of evaluation thus applies to situations that call for a summation and a summative role for evaluation.

WHO MAKES THE EVALUATIVE JUDGMENTS?

Judgments about the worth of a given evaluand or program should be made after analysis of the assembled evidence. The evidence can be of a qualitative or quantitative nature, or a combination of both. A study designed to assess the worth of a major educational policy used largely qualitative data obtained from schools by observation, interview and document analysis. The focus of the study was the policy's impact on school practice, and thus concentrated on its implementation across the school system.

The client for the findings was a government education committee for which a final report was prepared. In Example 1.2 a copy of the first page of this report is presented. The findings were presented as a discussion based on five objectives of the policy. The reporting strategy was to present a summary of the findings, and allow members of the committee to make their own judgments about the effectiveness and worth of the policy. This was done in recognition that different members of the committee and other readers would have different opinions of the relative importance of each of the policy objectives.

In this example, the evaluators:

- encouraged clients, in this case a committee, to make a judgment of worth;
- explicitly introduced the notion of values to the clients in the evaluation report.

Example 1.2 Evaluating the Curriculum and Standards Framework (CSF)

First page of final evaluation report

[Note that we have not included details of references here]
A key aspect of evaluation is making a judgment of the worth or merit of the policy or program under review. Kirkhart and Ruffolo believe that it is important to be explicit about the criteria being used to determine worth. There is also an associated issue of who makes the necessary judgments. While the onus of judgment is often on the evaluator, stakeholders are sometimes in a better position to determine the value of a given program.

Synthesis of the evaluation findings

Below, we lay out the more salient conclusions from the case studies, so that an evaluative judgment can be made. While we are prepared to make conclusions we prefer to leave the final judgment of the impact of this policy to the readers of this report. This is an acknowledgment of the fact that value judgments are relative. That is, what one stakeholder might value is likely to differ from that of another stakeholder.

The conclusions are organized around five themes. We believe that these themes provide a valid framework for making evaluative judgments. They were derived from the early stated policy documentation, from the time the CSF was released to schools. As such, they are explicit and independent of any one person's view of what the CSF should achieve. The themes also incorporate the facets about which the primary stakeholders expressed an interest.

The themes were:

- Adaptation at School Level;
- Selecting and Arranging the Curriculum;
- Assessment and Reporting;
- Accountability to the Community and to the System; and
- Policy–School Level Interaction.

In making a judgment about the worth of a program, there is a tendency to reduce the judgment to a single finding, to say that the object being evaluated is 'OK' or 'not much good'. Taking a line from the evaluation of products, some evaluators have urged that a single judgment can be made about educational programs. Our view is that the real world is more complex, and that most policies or programs need to be considered on several dimensions. This is the position taken here. Judgments could be made for each theme on the basis of the summary presented. If a final single judgment of the worth of the CSF is to be made, it will depend on a stakeholder's valuing of the relative importance of the policy themes.

In this case the report formed the basis of a vigorous debate about the impact of the CSF policy at committee level (Owen et al. 1996). This example suggests that evaluators, in addition to undertaking empirical work, need to engage with clients to determine on what basis the evaluation should proceed. For example, clients and evaluators might enter into discussion, in advance of any evidence collection, as to who, or what group, is to make a judgment about the worth of the program under review. In some instances, the client of an evaluation is more than happy to let the evaluator do so. But in other cases, the client prefers to take this responsibility. The bottom line is that, in studies that use the logic of evaluation, a judgment of worth must be made by someone.

The principles of evaluation logic can be applied to a variety of circumstances over and above those related to determining the worth of a product, policy or program. This application of evaluation logic can be used to develop frameworks for personnel performance appraisals. This usually involves deriving criteria from job descriptions, and the collection of evidence from key informants, such as the supervisor of the person being appraised, or from a range of respondents who are familiar with the work of the person.

The logic can also be applied in the management of evaluation. For example, the selection of a consultant was a major task for a committee responsible for the evaluation of a community housing program. Based on the criteria set out in the evaluation brief, a protocol was developed to assess the worth of all consultant groups which had forwarded a tender to undertake the study. This involved the development of a scoring grid that led to the ranking of all applications by committee members, and the selection of the consultant with the top score to undertake the evaluation.

EXPANDING THE INFLUENCE OF EVALUATIVE INQUIRY

At this point, you might assume that *all* evaluations can be based on the evaluation logic we have just outlined. This is not the case. While there is obviously a need for program managers to know whether or not their program 'works', they often need alternative information, such as what to do if their program is not working.

This has been long recognized among the evaluator community. At an International Evaluation Conference in Vancouver in 1995, Michael Scriven distinguished between evaluation based on the logic just outlined, and 'what evaluators do'. This implied that evaluators undertake studies we will refer to as *evaluative inquiry* that respond to a range of information needs among decision-makers, of which the establishment of a program's worth was but one.

House (1993) suggests that evaluative inquiry consists of:

> collecting data, including relevant variables and standards, resolving inconsistencies in the values, clarifying misunderstandings and misrepresentations, rectifying false facts and factual assumptions, distinguishing between wants and needs, identifying all relevant dimensions of merit, finding appropriate measures for these dimensions, weighting the dimensions, validating the standards, and arriving at an evaluative conclusion (p. 8).

Evaluative inquiry can focus on one or more aspects of policy or program delivery—development, implementation or impact. Consistent with House, we take the view that evaluative inquiry should respond to questions of concern to identified clients, and that the findings should be framed to assist decision-making about the program under review.

Typical scenarios that are amenable to evaluative inquiry include the following:

1. A philanthropic agency has funded an after-school recreation program as part of an initiative to reduce juvenile crime. After several years, an evaluation is commissioned to see whether the program has been effective.
2. A new community center is being planned. An analysis of the needs of the community, including population information, availability of other facilities and a feasibility study, is put in train.
3. Weekly and monthly measures of the performance of major programs administered by a state government department are mandated by the state treasury.

You may be aware that Scenario 1 poses questions one associates with traditional evaluation questions such as:

- How good is this program? and,
- Did the program work?

As we have discussed, evaluative inquiry is concerned with these questions. But it is also concerned with others, such as:

- What is needed?
- How can we design a program to meet these needs?
- What is happening in this program?
- How is the program performing on a continuous basis?
- How could we improve this program? and,
- How could we repeat the success of this program elsewhere?

The expanded definition of evaluative inquiry based on these notions is presented in Figure 1.2, in which evaluation work based on judgment of worth is shown as a subset of a broader endeavor.

Figure 1.2 Evaluation definitions

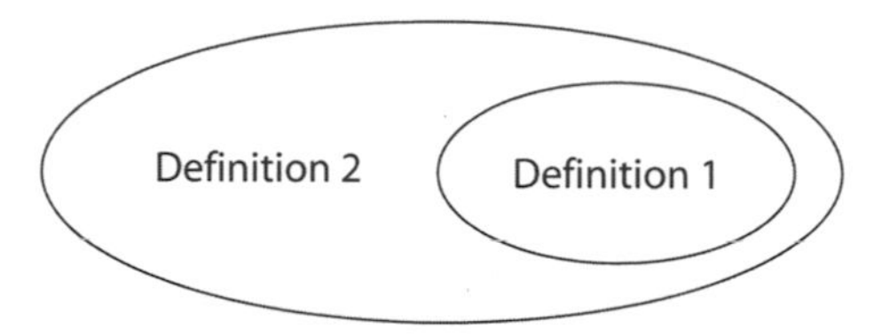

Definition 1: Evaluation as the judgment of worth of a program.
Definition 2: Evaluation as the production of knowledge based on systematic inquiry to assist decision-making about a program.

Evaluative inquiry undertaken in conjunction with Scenarios 2 and 3 above are amenable to some of these questions. In this and following chapters we make more explicit some of the assumptions underlying evaluation practice, with a view to defining what we mean by 'evaluative inquiry'. Thus, this book takes an expanded perspective of evaluation compared to one concerned with the judgment of program worth. It also focuses, not only on the practice of 'professional' evaluators, but also on the contribution and roles of managers, program providers, funders, recipients and others who have legitimate interests in the evaluation process.

EVALUATION IN THE CONTEXT OF DECISION-MAKING

The discussion above implies that evaluators need to expand their epistemological and methodological repertoire rather than relying on the logic of evaluation as the basis for their work. In addition, if we accept the emphasis on responding to the knowledge needs of stakeholders, it follows that evaluators cannot work in a vacuum. They must develop strategies that enable them to discover these needs and decide how empirical inquiry can be used to determine answers to the questions that stakeholders pose. These strategies can be thought of as involving negotiation between program stakeholders and evaluators, with a view to coming to a common understanding of how the remainder of the evaluation process will proceed.

And, if we are serious about evaluation affecting decision-making by stakeholders, we need also to attend to the use of findings. Thus, evaluators need to develop skills related to the dissemination of the knowledge that is produced.

These ideas have been taken up by a subset of the evaluation community and gained prominence over the past decade. For example, studies in the United States and elsewhere have encouraged organizations to be engaged in internally-based evaluation with a view to encouraging change and improvement (Owen et al. 1994; Preskill & Torres 1996). We have also seen an increase in the influence of theorists with a special interest in the importance of interactive links between clients and evaluators, such as Michael Patton in the United States, Murray Saunders in Great Britain, and Bradley Cousins in Canada.

In summary, evaluation involves much more than designing a sound empirical study. A more inclusive list of the work of evaluators includes negotiating the key issues for a study, attending to ethical considerations, collecting and analyzing evidence, disseminating to audiences, and assisting with the implementation of findings.

This is summarized in the description of evaluative inquiry as the processes of:

- negotiating an evaluation plan;
- implementing an evaluation design to produce findings;
- disseminating to identified audiences for use in:
  - describing or understanding an evaluand, or
  - making judgments or decisions related to that evaluand.

EVALUATION FINDINGS

Within the framework above, the notion of *findings* from empirical inquiry is central. While we will come back to this notion later in this book, it is worth completing this chapter with a brief discussion of what we mean by the term.

Findings encompass the following:

- *Evidence* The data and other information which has been collected during the evaluation.
- *Conclusions* The synthesis of data and information. These are the meanings those involved in the evaluation make through the synthesis of data. This involves evaluators in data display, data reduction and verification processes.
- *Judgments* Placing value on conclusions. Criteria are applied to the conclusions stating that the program is 'good' or 'bad', or that the results are 'positive', 'in the direction desired', or 'below expectations'.
- *Recommendations* These are suggested courses of action, advice to policy-makers, program managers or providers about what to do in the light of the evidence and conclusions.

Our view is that *all* evaluative inquiry involves collecting evidence and making conclusions. However, there will be variations from study to study in the degree to which findings incorporate the making of judgments or recommendations. This will be illustrated in the case examples used to illustrate key points throughout this book.

CONCLUSION

We would like you to keep in mind the distinction between evaluation based on the logic of evaluation and evaluative inquiry, as defined above. However, there is also something to be said for using terms that have familiarity and can be employed easily in discussion. Thus, we will use interchangeably the terms 'evaluative inquiry' and 'evaluation' with the proviso that the term 'evaluation' takes on the broader connotation as outlined above.

The remainder of the book is designed to assist you in making sense of the role of an evaluator who is willing to work within a framework of evaluative inquiry. Making the leap from the logic of evaluation to evaluative inquiry greatly enlarges both the conceptual knowledge base required of a student of evaluation, and the ways in which the evaluator might work. The evaluator must have a firm conceptual grasp of these ideas in order to make sound decisions about how an evaluative inquiry should be pursued in a given scenario. The first element of this knowledge base is to explore the range of evaluands that an evaluator might encounter, and this is discussed in Chapter 2.

REFERENCES

Fournier, D. M. (1995). Establishing evaluative conclusions: A distinction between general and working logic. *New Directions for Program Evaluation*, 68 (Winter 1995), 15–32.

House, E. R. (1993). *Professional Evaluation: Social Impact and Political Consequences*. Thousand Oaks, CA: Sage.

Kirkhart, K. E. and Ruffolo, M. C. (1993). Value bases of case management. *Evaluation and Program Planning*, 16, 55–65.

Owen, J. M. and Downtown, A. P. (1990). *Towards Effective Conference Design*. Centre for Program Evaluation, The University of Melbourne, Australia.

Owen, J. M., Lambert, F. C. and Stringer, W. S. (1994). Acquiring knowledge of implementation and change: Essential for program evaluators? *Knowledge: Creation, Diffusion, Utilization*, 15(3), 273–294.

Owen, J. M., Meyer, H. and Livingston, J. (1996). *School Responses to the Curriculum and Standards Framework*. Carlton, Australia: Victorian Board of Studies.

Preskill, H. and Torres, R. T. (1996). *From Evaluation to Evaluative Inquiry for Organizational Learning*. Paper presented at the annual meeting of the American Evaluation Association, Atlanta, GA, November 1996.

Scriven, M. (1971). Evaluating Educational Programs. In F. G. Caro (ed.), *Readings in Evaluation Research*. New York: Russell Sage Foundation.

2 The Nature of Interventions: What We Evaluate

In Chapter 1 we introduced some key ideas about evaluation that have emerged over time, and introduced a working definition of what we mean by evaluation. We also put forward a view of evaluation as complementary to, and supportive of, the development and provision of effective and responsive public and private sector interventions.

All programmatic interventions cost money and resources. In a civil society it is incumbent on public and not-for-profit providers to ensure that policies, support and administrative programs and other resources designed to improve the social condition are as effective and efficient as possible. This means responsive program planning, attention to implementation, and checking to see that program intentions have been translated into outcomes. Evaluative inquiry has a potential role at all stages of program provision.

The need for effective and efficient program planning takes place against a backdrop of governments of all political persuasions providing services in a time of economic constraint, and an increased concern among communities that money be spent wisely. One particular concern is that funds allocated to disadvantaged community groups are actually spent 'on the ground' in ways that directly benefit those for whom they have been earmarked. For example, in countries such as Canada and Australia, there has been concern that funds designed to provide health and welfare support for indigenous peoples have been used inefficiently, on poorly conceived interventions which have made little impact on the well-being of the recipients.

Evaluators should thus be concerned with understanding the nature of interventions or evaluands, such as:

- their internal structure and functioning;
- constraints that shape design and delivery; and

- societal factors that influence the development of evaluands, how evaluands themselves change over time, and how, in turn the evaluand contributes to social change (Shadish et al. 1991, p. 37).

Taken together, these aspects attend to program design and implementation as well as the links between the evaluand and the context in which it is set. This reminds us that social and educational interventions do not exist in a vacuum, and that evaluators need to be mindful of the influence of context when planning studies and providing advice to policy and program developers.

There is often uncertainty about the meaning of terms used to describe different evaluands. We need to have a working understanding of types of interventions and associated concepts, so that a common 'evaluator language' can be built up to serve as a sound base for exploration of key issues. So the next section provides some shared definitions. Then, a more meaningful discussion can be advanced about ways in which evaluation can be used to develop, review or improve an evaluand, the 'object' of an evaluation.

It is also important that the evaluator and others interested in the findings of an evaluation are clear about the focus of a given evaluative inquiry. While this might sound trite, experience shows that being absolutely unambiguous about the *what* of evaluation is essential if the evaluation is to go forward to answer other fundamental questions, such as why the evaluation is being conducted.

OBJECTS OF AN EVALUATION

Likely objects for evaluation include:

- policies;
- programs;
- products; and
- individuals.

Each is discussed in turn below.

Policies

Policies can be considered as the most pervasive form of social intervention. All government departments produce policies: vast amounts of time and energy are expended in their development, and public policy is an essential topic for students of governance and organizational change. Yet, despite the hundreds of books devoted to policy, it is difficult to find a satisfactory definition in the social science literature. Bauer (1968) suggests that:

> various labels are applied to decisions and actions we take, depending in general on the breadth of their implications. If they are trivial and repetitive and demand little cognition, they may be called routine actions. If they are somewhat more complex, have wider ramifications, and demand more thought, we may refer to them as tactical decisions. For those which have the widest ramifications and the longest time perspective, and which generally require the most information and contemplation, we tend to reserve the term 'policy' (p. 14).

Policies tend to be the domain of strategic planners; those at the 'center' of systemic and organizational arrangements.

A scan of the literature suggests three domains of policy influence:

- legislative policy;
- large-scale policy; and
- local policy.

Legislative policy comes in the form of a government bill or parliamentary Act. It enables the allocation of funds for major initiatives by parliament, congress or similar bodies, such as a government executive. For example, a national legislature passed the Supported Accommodation Assistance Act, a policy that enabled the provision of accommodation and other benefits to those regarded as homeless. The Act sets out in detail the objectives of the policy and how it will be administered.

Large-scale policy provides direction for interventions that are implemented across a system of providers under the same organizational umbrella. For example, a government department initiated a drug education policy and guidelines for implementation that was disseminated to every school in a state education system. Over a period of two years, schools were required to implement the policy with support from consultants provided by the department.

Local policy provides direction for implementation across a single site. For example, a corporation could adopt a learning and development policy, or a university could implement a policy on the regular appraisal of administrative staff.

It is evident that policy scholars experience some difficulty in defining what is meant by the term 'policy'. Looking at the development of policy across institutions such as Congress, State legislatures and higher education accreditation boards in the United States (Guba 1984) developed the following eight perspectives. Policy is:

- an assertion of intents or goals;
- a governing body's 'standing decisions' by which it regulates, controls, promotes, services and otherwise influences matters within its sphere of authority;
- a guide to discretionary action;
- a strategy undertaken to solve or ameliorate some problem;
- sanctioned behavior, formally through authoritative decisions, or informally through expectations and acceptance, established over time;
- a norm of conduct, characterized by consistency and regularity, in some substantive action area;
- the output of the policy-making system: the cumulative effect of all the actions, decisions and behaviors of the millions of people who work in bureaucracies. It occurs, takes place and is made at every point in the policy cycle, from agenda-setting to policy impact. As such, policy is an analytical category.
- the impact of the policy-making and policy-implementing system as it is experienced by the client.

Kahn (1969) suggests that policies are 'standing plans'—guides to future decision-making that are intended to shape those decisions. Decisions must be consistent with a goal, an integral part of the policy documentation. A policy is a general guide to action, an overarching statement that includes this goal and guiding principles for an intervention. According to Guba and Kahn, policy documentation thus has some characteristics in common with strategic plans—for example, the inclusion of goals. However, most policies are more general than strategic plans—for example, they are less likely to specify the means by which the ends are to be attained. This implies that a policy provides general directions for action but in itself does not prescribe a course of action.

We expect that programs would be developed which are consistent with the direction of the policy in a given area of concern. For example, a government's policy about welfare housing might translate into different programs in different locations. This suggests that policy is at least once removed from specifications of action, and so evaluations designed to determine the effects of policy must take this into account.

However, there is a trend for policies to be specified in a way that blurs the distinction between policy and strategic planning. We suggest that contemporary policy should be:

- *evidence informed*—based on the best available systematic information about the problem the policy is being designed to ameliorate;
- *change focused*—takes into account the latest research on effective change and implementation theories;
- *inclusive*—recognizes the interests of a range of policy stakeholders;
- *strategic*—contributes to the overall mission and vision of the auspicing department or agency;
- *causal*—pays attention to the links between delivery and outcomes;
- *joined up*—works across departmental or sectoral boundaries;
- *realistic*—takes into account the realities faced by those responsible for implementation;
- *flexible*—can be applied in a range of settings; and
- *outcomes orientated*—focuses on delivering benefits to policy clients (Owen & St Leger 2004).

Two major investigatory activities related to policy have emerged in the social science literature. These are policy analysis and policy research.

- *Policy analysis* is concerned with issues such as giving an account of the development of a policy, the explication of the choices that faced the policy-maker, and the assumptions made and values employed in making choices between alternatives. Much of what passes as policy analysis could be thought of as reflective, often done in retrospect, relying on secondary data, and directed towards an understanding of policy development *per se*, rather than towards the improvement of a specific policy initiative.
- *Policy research* (which, in the context of this book, might be renamed *policy evaluation*) involves the determination of the policy impact for the direct and timely use by those responsible for a policy intervention. Johnson (1975) suggests that policy evaluation could operate in a range of modes, from description of the impact of a policy, through explanation of why patterns of impact occur, through to criticism of the policy direction. The systematic collection and analysis of evidence is seen as the first step to scientific criticism of policy.

Programs

Smith (1989) defines a program as: 'a set of planned activities directed toward bringing about specified change(s) in an identified and identifiable audience' (p. 47).

This suggests that a program has two essential components:

- a documented plan; and
- action consistent with the documentation contained in the plan.

A program can be thought of as an intentional effort at change which, in addition to its effect on participants, may have secondary effects on the context within which the program is located—for example, an organization or more diverse socio-cultural setting.

Figure 2.1 Program components

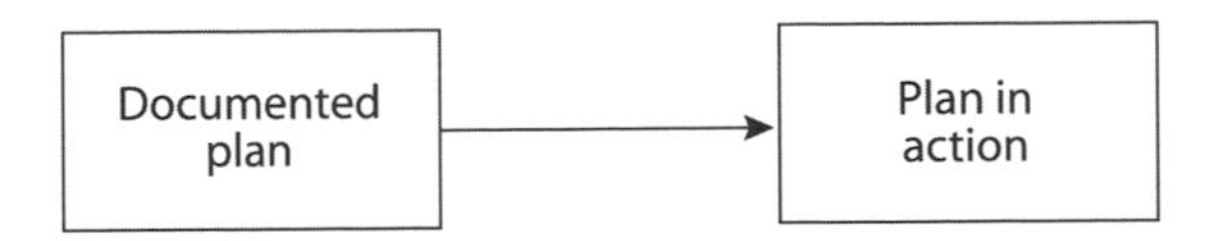

Formal evaluation language speaks of a 'theory of action' or a program logic that specifies linkages between various components of implementation, and between them and one or more outcomes. (Much more will be said about program logic later in this book.) Effective planning rests on the assumption that those responsible have sufficient skill to codify solutions to the problem that the program addresses. The plan must be outlined in a format that can be disseminated and understood by those with an interest in the impact of the program—for example, program deliverers, and those who are the intended beneficiaries.

Program levels

Programs can be planned and presented at several levels.

The broadest is the *mega* level—at the level of the head of a government department's office or the boardroom of a private company. This is sometimes described as the *corporate level*. At this level planning is likely to be in terms of overall economic or social impact. A second level is *macro* planning, which may be the responsibility of divisions, regions or groups within an organization. The third level is the *micro* level, the responsibility of work units or individuals. The degree and emphasis on planning which takes place at each of these levels varies from setting to setting.

The level of a program can have implications for approaches to evaluation. There may be different concerns at each level of an organization about a given intervention. Evaluators must be sensitive to these needs when designing evaluations intended to be responsive to audiences at each level.

Example 2.1 Evaluation agendas of stakeholders at different levels of provision

A training policy was developed to provide people with skills to work in the area of intellectual disability. The resulting course of study was produced by a central curriculum agency and taught in 16 higher education colleges across an education system. Within this framework, different evaluation agendas can be imagined that are related to decisions about the intervention. For example:

- *Mega level*: The Treasury Department, with the total cost of the program in mind, may wish to know whether the course, taken over all colleges, and over a period of time, is providing adequate graduates to staff intellectual disability centers.
- *Macro level*: The curriculum agency may wish to know whether the curriculum is actually providing graduates with the skills needed to perform on the job. This evaluation may be motivated by a need to revise the curriculum.
- *Micro level*: Staff responsible for the course in one of the colleges may be unhappy with the way they are delivering the course. This evaluation may be motivated by a wish to fine-tune the delivery to make the teaching more effective and to use staff time more efficiently.

Different questions need to be answered at each level. A combination of the level and the concerns of audiences at each level implies that the agenda of evaluative inquiry would be different in each case.

While it is possible for corporations to develop mega-level programs, they are most evident in the role of government departments in areas such as health, welfare and education. Mega-level programs are sometimes called 'Program Areas'.

Example 2.2 Programs in community services

A state government agency responsible for social welfare organized its services through six Program Areas:

- Community Support;
- Family and Children's Support Service;
- Alternative Accommodation and Care;

- Youth Services;
- Intellectual Disabilities Services; and
- Health and Community Care.

The annual budgets for these Program Areas ranged from $62 million to $480 million in the financial year 2000/01. Each of these Programs was delivered through offices spread across regions of the state.

In some organizations the term 'Division' rather than 'Program Area' is used. A policy statement is often developed for the work of a Division or Program Area, which includes objectives, either implicitly or explicitly stated, designed to guide the work in each Division.

Example 2.3 Divisions as Programs

An Office of Corrections divided its operations into Divisions, one of which was the Division of Prisons. An analysis of the operational plan of the Division of Prisons revealed that its mission was to:

- manage and administer the sentence proposed by the courts;
- provide sufficient security to minimize danger of offenders inflicting harm on themselves, other inmates, staff or the public;
- meet the humane, medical and health care needs of offenders;
- assist offenders to develop and adopt acceptable behavior patterns; and
- assist offenders to become responsible citizens through education, training, social development and work experience.

It is interesting to note that while the Division was responsible for more specific interventions of a smaller scale, its main concern was the day-to-day administration of prisons across the state.

Day (1990, p. 205) assisted this Office of Corrections to develop monitoring indicators to gauge the impact of the Division of Prisons. This was in response to the need of Office of Corrections management to have access to information to account for the funds spent. At the time, there was a heavy emphasis in government agencies on developing and using appropriate outcome measures, generally in the form of a series of indicators of performance. Despite this emphasis, it is now difficult to find exemplary cases where Program performance measures are routinely used in mega program evaluation.

Program Areas or Divisions are obviously at the mega end of the levels of program planning and delivery introduced earlier in this chapter. Recent observers have noted the difficulty of undertaking evaluation work at this level because the goals are often broad and there is difficulty in attribution, but in some jurisdictions this is precisely the level at which evaluation activity is focused. This is due to the fact that, at this level, budgetary appropriations become manifest, and government priorities are turned into practice.

Example 2.4 The Program Assessment Rating Tool (PART)

In the United States, the Office of Management and Budget in the General Accounting Office has developed the PART tool to monitor the impact of Program Areas for the Federal Government. The process is designed to assess the quality of design and planning, rate the management of the Program, and rate the quality of the performance indicators used by the agency in monitoring progress, as well at the results which are achieved based on these indicators.

At the next level down from mega programs, we can think of macro (hereafter 'Big P') programs. These can be thought of as specific interventions, with a tighter link between objectives, implementation and outcomes that in the case of mega programs (or Program Areas). A key aspect of a macro program is take-up at multiple sites. In the case of the drug education policy discussed earlier in this chapter, a macro program was developed with clear and explicit guidelines about implementation for all schools. One issue regarding implementation of macro programs is the degree to which adaptations in program intent at individual sites is acceptable.

One could think of the implementation of an individual school's drug education strategy as the micro-level program in this context. We will sometimes refer to programs at this level as 'little p' programs.

It is clear that there are often links between macro and micro programs, and studies involving both levels are currently one of the major methodological challenges for evaluators. Evaluations of this type are known as multi-level multi-site studies.

Program typologies

Many programs are described as *social interventions*. They are provided to the community by government or not-for-profit agencies on the basis of 'non-market' criteria, in areas such as welfare, health and education. A review of social interventions suggests that we need to extend the definition of a program introduced earlier in this chapter to encompass a more extensive range of program interventions. At one level, we can distinguish between programs designed to produce an end result by influencing behavior, and those that are designed to satisfy a need by providing a product or a service.

Extending this distinction and incorporating the contributions of Funnell and Lenne (1989), five specific types of intervention can be identified:

- *Educational programs*—which emphasize the acquisition of information, skills and attitudes (ISA), typically provided through formal learning settings by institutions such as schools, colleges and the like. Examples include:
  - a reading program at an adult education center;
  - an in-house training program for child protection workers.
- *Advisory programs*—such as communication and mass education programs for the public. The receptiveness of the target group is dependent not only on the quality of the intervention, but also on the credibility of those who have the responsibility to 'sell' the product. This is the motivation behind employing people with high public profiles to encourage change of behavior of the clients. Examples include:
  - a health promotion program designed to improve the eating habits and general well-being of the citizens in a targeted region or city. An example is an Australian advertising campaign which used well-known football players as role models;
  - a publicity program encouraging people to visit a region or area of natural beauty—for example, the Lakes District in England or the Banff-Jasper Parkway in Canada.
- *Regulatory programs*—which influence behavior through a process of deterrence. While the likelihood of incurring a penalty is believed to have an effect on behavior, recent studies suggest that the perceived chance of being detected is the more powerful influence. Examples include:
  - the implementation of measures to reduce the incidence of alcohol-induced accidents on the roads—for example, enforcement of blood alcohol standards for drivers;

- the enforcement of fishing regulations which deter professional fisherman and weekend anglers from taking fish under a given size, with a view to ensuring an adequate supply of the species in the longer term.

- *Case management programs*—where individual objectives are set for each case within an overall program framework. The 'case' may be an individual or a group within an organization. A feature of case management is that a plan must be developed for each case. Examples include:
  - a systematic set of rehabilitation procedures designed for an individual worker injured on the job;
  - the development and implementation of case plans for children needing foster care because of family dislocation.
- *Product or service provision*—examples of which include:
  - the provision of meals and other forms of support for the elderly who are unable to fully fend for themselves while remaining within their own residences;
  - the provision of a power line to an isolated community in a valley not presently covered by the national electricity grid.

Some services may be used as an individual pleases—for example, facilities in a local park. Others may be available according to the status of the individual in a social system—for example, access to child minding services may only be available to families with children within a given age range. Still others, such as meals for elderly citizens, may be made available as a result of the professional judgment of a social worker. Even for programs that directly provide a tangible product or service, there are often consequences beyond the immediate intended outcomes. The provision of a power line to an isolated community, for example, may have economic, agricultural and labor implications that should be considered in the decision to go ahead with the project. The program planner should anticipate these effects and monitor the expected and unexpected outcomes of the intervention.

In the real world a program might use a combination of two or more typologies. For example, a program to reduce the road toll in the state of Victoria, Australia, has used a combination of advisory and regulatory interventions. The advisory component includes a range of mass communication strategies, including billboard displays, television and radio advertisements, and sponsorship. The regulatory component includes the use of speed traps and 'booze buses', which are randomly deployed on the state's roads. While these strategies have been introduced progressively over the years, and their sophistication has increased, the state has had a long-term commitment to safer roads with marked success. From a peak of 1064 persons killed on Victorian roads in 1970, the road toll had fallen to 397 in 2002 (Department of Transport and Regional Services 2003).

The implications for evaluators who are asked to determine the impact of programs that fall into each typology should be clear. In general, evaluation designs, which involve decisions about data collection and analysis, must take into account the nature of the program being studied. The typology provides a degree of structure for evaluators in the sense that programs within a given typology should be amenable to similar, if not the same, evaluation designs.

A key issue in many impact evaluations is causality—the determination of attribution. In other words, the determination of the degree to which program implementation leads to the desired outcomes. Another challenge for evaluators is to develop evaluation designs for programs that have several components, as is the case for the road toll reduction program just discussed. Here, in addition to attribution, the evaluator may be asked to estimate the contribution of each of the components to the desired outcomes.

Specificity of program plans

The creation of a program involves a planning process. Moving from planning to program development means converting value choices into concrete directions for action by choosing among alternatives and allocating resources to achieve defined goals.

Expectations about the specificity of program documentation, and hence prescriptions for action, vary. We have seen that programs can be classified along two dimensions, according to:

- level (mega, macro, micro); and
- type (educational, advisory, regulatory, case management, service/ product provision).

One could think of the development of a three-by-five matrix within which an evaluator could classify an intervention of interest. This may be helpful if you are asked to think about undertaking an evaluation, because locating a given program in such a matrix almost certainly will reduce the possible decisions about how an evaluation should proceed.

As a rule, as one moves from mega to micro, the specificity of planning increases. While a regional or school district science program may be written in general terms (macro/educational), a six-week science curriculum unit is likely to be more detailed (micro/ educational). One question that arises is: What level of detail is adequate in order for those involved to know what the program is really about?

Leithwood (1981) suggests that a curriculum unit would be adequately specified if the program plan contained coherent information on the following dimensions:

- platform;
- objectives;
- student entry behaviors;
- assessment tools and procedures;
- instructional materials;
- learner experiences;
- teaching strategies;
- content; and
- time or length of the unit.

Educators and even those with limited educational background can readily understand most of these dimensions. The possible exception is 'platform'. Leithwood defines platform as:

> patterns of implicit and explicit beliefs and assumptions accepted as the bases about what to include in and exclude from a curriculum . . . Such platforms are the product of interactions between a developer's value systems on the one hand, and information about society, culture, learners, the learning process and the nature of knowledge on the other (p. 26).

The inclusion of platform or a rationale in the program specification reinforces what was said before: that programs do not exist in a vacuum, but are a response to a variety of influences, including that of perceived need in a given context.

Not all programs may need the degree of specification suggested by Leithwood. For example, a planned intervention designed to save homes and gardens due to cliff erosion along the southern Californian coast, which could be classified as a macro/service provision program, may require little more than a rationale, a set of intentions (goals or objectives), details about resource requirements, and a statement of how the program is to proceed. Some program plans may also incorporate an evaluative component—for example, variables and indicators for monitoring program implementation and impact. This reinforces what was said in the introduction to this chapter: that we should view evaluation as something that is not divorced from program provision.

In practice, we find that even these minimum specification requirements are often not met, that many operating programs have no statement that outlines the essential features of the intervention. Program planners often seem to have difficulty in developing links between ends and means, and causes and effects. A major issue is the development of meaningful goals.

Our experience is that writing specific goals up front is very difficult. The 'real' goals of a program often emerge during the 'first round' or trial of a program. A realistic approach to specifying goals is therefore to work backwards from what developers see as plausible program achievements as the basis for setting its true goals.

Now that we have some idea of what is meant by an intervention, several possibilities arise as to the focus and issues for an evaluation of a specific program. One possibility is the degree of internal consistency between the program plan and action. A key issue could be: To what extent is the implementation consistent with the plan for implementation? The evaluation might identify problems, if any, associated with the effective delivery of the program. Alternatively, one might ask about the extent to which the outcomes were consistent with program goals.

Understanding what is meant by an intervention in a generic sense enables us to focus in on the specific object under evaluative review. An entire program could be considered if we wanted to know if it was effective. It could be, however, that the evaluators are asked to focus on one component of the program. For example, invoking the Leithwood framework, the science department in a school might want answers to the following questions about the implementation of the unit:

- Are the teaching strategies working?
- Is the time allocated to this unit long enough?

In this case, the evaluation focuses on two components of the program: teaching strategies and time allocation. This means that the evaluator can devote evaluation resources to the objects of concern to the decision-makers.

In summary, a proposed intervention must have some direction to actually be considered as a program. At a minimum there must be an implicit direction of action that someone has in mind. Invariably, making this explicit helps the developer to think in causal terms and aids implementation. Documenting what is to happen or has happened also makes the program public, an essential condition to justify the resources devoted to program planning and implementation.

Having discussed various levels of programmatic interventions it is reasonable to ask questions about the links between them.

Shadish et al. (1991) and others put the situation in the United States in the following way:

> Policy expresses intentions about the kind of executive and legislative actions that have priority. Policy gives guiding assumptions and goals for many programs, and may be formally codified or informally expressed by policy makers in speeches, agendas, or expressions of support or opposition. Programs are administrative umbrellas for distributing funds under a policy. Programs rarely turn over entirely . . . They are mostly changeable at the margins, so a summative evaluation of a program will rarely if ever result in a complete program replacement . . . Programs are not homogeneous. They consist of locally implemented projects where service delivery occurs . . . Projects can differ widely in character within the same program, because they are implemented under a national tradition of local control, service providers have discretion in the services they implement, and needs and demands change from place to place and over time at the same place. Like programs, projects have great staying power (p. 107).

The closest to our micro level or 'little p' program in Shadish's terms is the notion of a 'project'. However, an important distinction is that 'little p' programs do not necessarily have to fit under a broader umbrella—that is, they do not have to be part of a Big P program, as Shadish and his colleagues assert. This may have to do with the nature of public sector funding in different countries. In Britain or Australia, for example, it is not uncommon for funding support to be sought or provided directly to local agencies to develop and trial a small-scale program without reference to a larger administrative umbrella—in effect, there is more often a direct link between policy and little p program provision. This reminds us of the assertion made at the beginning of this chapter, that program provision needs to be understood within the social and political context. In this case there are obviously national level differences which impinge on how social and educational policy and programs are delivered.

Products

Another class of objects of evaluation are *products*—for example, a software computer package, or a technical manual used in on-the-job training. We have come across the evaluation of a product in the example of evaluating breakfast cereals presented in Chapter 1. You will have noted that the approach taken there was to provide comparative data on a set of criteria, and then to present or display these data to make recommendations about the 'best buy'. This approach could be used to make decisions about the adoption of resources—for example, the choice of a given textbook for use in a specific educational program. In this case it is important that the criteria used take into account the needs of the students and the nature of the curriculum within which the text will be used.

Product evaluation provides a basis within which the logic of evaluation can be invoked and transferred to program evaluation. However, as we saw in Chapter 1, the extrapolation from product to program evaluation introduces a set of complexities for the evaluator, such as requiring the context of program provision to be taken into account.

Individuals

We have come to accept the need for evidence about the performance of individuals to be collected and used in corporate and social systems. The most prevalent terms now in use are *performance assessment* and *performance appraisal*. Assessment is generally used to describe the achievement of students in formal learning settings such as a college or university, while appraisal is usually associated with the performance of professionals or employees.

Key features in the reform of assessment and appraisal include:

- the conceptual separation of assessment from testing and the encouragement by authorities of an assessment rather than a testing culture;
- an increased understanding of the various uses and reporting of assessment (diagnosis/grading) and implications for the ways in which evidence about individuals is assembled;
- a concern for authentic methods of assessing the actual achievements of individuals;
- an enhanced role for instructor observation and judgment in the assessment of competencies; and
- the development of innovative ways of setting up assessment frameworks—for example, student profiles that enable the progress of students to be indicated.

These are key issues in setting up acceptable performance assessment regimes for use in assessment and appraisal systems.

Evidence of attainment can be used to rank or grade individuals for purposes of certification or selection—for example, across the school–college interface, or as the basis for employment or individual diagnosis and improvement.

Assessment information can also be used in conjunction with program or policy evaluation, particularly studies of impact. Typically, we are interested in determining whether the program makes a difference to the performance or attainment of those for whom it is intended. If this information is used to make decisions *about the program*, then this is seen as a legitimate part of program evaluation.

However, if the emphasis on information collection about individuals is to decide on aspects such as promotion, reallocation or dismissal, the process is more appropriately thought of as assessment or performance appraisal. This is a most important distinction that must be understood by budding program evaluators.

REFERENCES

Bauer, R. A. (1968). The study of policy formation. In R. A. Bauer and K. J. Gergen (eds), *The Study of Policy Formation*. London: The Free Press.

Day, N. A. (1990). 'Performance Indicators in Custodial and Community Programs.' Unpublished paper, Centre for Program Evaluation, The University of Melbourne.

Department of Transport and Regional Services (2003). *Road Crash Data and Rates: Australian States and Territories*. Australian Transport Safety Bureau.

Funnell, S. and Lenne, B. (1989). *A Typology of Public Sector Programs*. Paper presented at the Annual Meeting of the American Evaluation Association, November, San Francisco.

Guba, E. G. (1984). *The Impact of Various Definitions of Policy on the Nature and Outcomes of Policy Analysis*. Paper presented at the Annual Meeting of the American Educational Research Association, New Orleans, LA.

Johnson, R. W. (1975). Research objectives for policy analysis. In K. M. Dolbeare (ed), *Public Policy Evaluation: Sage Yearbook in Politics and Public Policy* (Vol. II, pp. 75–92). Beverly Hills, CA: Sage.

Kahn, A. J. (1969). *Theory and Practice of Social Planning*. New York: Russell Sage Foundation.

Leithwood, K. (1981). Dimensions of curriculum innovation. *Journal of Curriculum Studies*, 13, 26–37.

Owen, J. M. and St Leger, P. (2004). *Evaluating Policy: Trends and Issues*. Workshop presented at the Annual conference of the Australasian Evaluation Society, Adelaide.

Shadish, W. R., Cook, T. D. and Leviton, L. C. (1991). *Foundations of Program Evaluation*. Newbury Park: Sage.

Smith, M. E. (1989) *Evaluability Assessment: A Practical Approach*. Norwell, MA: Kluwer.

Focusing Evaluative Inquiry: Evaluation Forms and Approaches

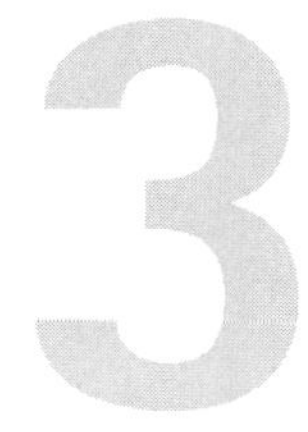

Over the past two decades theorists have put forward a range of evaluation models. A model can be thought of as a prescription for undertaking an evaluation, based on certain theoretical assumptions. The number of models proliferated as more social scientists entered the evaluation arena and attempts were made to classify them in terms of elements such as assumptions, methodology, and extent of involvement of stakeholders (Stufflebeam & Webster 1983).

Despite these attempts, we have found that many graduate students and commissioners of evaluation were confused about the relationship between a model and the solution to practical work-related problems. As one of our students, Susan Day, pointed out, what appeared to be missing from the evaluation literature was a framework that would make sense of this situation from the point of view of practitioners (Day 1991). To remedy this we developed a 'meta-model', consisting of five *Evaluation Forms*, within which some of the more important models or Approaches (as we shall call them) can be located. The Forms are designed to address the 'why' question in evaluation. Why an evaluation is being commissioned is of fundamental importance to both stakeholders and evaluators. Addressing the why question encourages evaluators to seek clarity about the knowledge needs of clients and sharpens up thinking about how this knowledge can be generated.

The notions of 'Form' and 'Approach' provide an epistemological framework for understanding the breadth of evaluative inquiry. For each Form there is a cluster of existing well-known Approaches that have elements in common. The Forms point to a range of roles for evaluative inquiry. This view is consistent with the comment of a noted evaluator that the 'world of evaluation has grown larger than the boundaries of formative and summative evaluation, though this distinction remains important and useful' (Patton 1996). So let us examine each of the Forms. At this stage we wish merely to sketch their connection to evaluation Approaches. In later chapters we provide information about the Approaches within each Form, and further expand the framework is by discussing implications for data management—the collection and analysis of evidence.

The notion of Form is an attempt at simplification while at the same time acknowledging the complexity of the field. For many users of this book, the selection of a Form will suffice in planning an evaluation study—that is, the planner need not delve into the differences between Approaches within the selected Form. Others who see the need to use a more refined conceptual base for a study would choose not only the Form, but also an Approach within that Form, as the basis for their investigation.

THE 'WHY' QUESTION AND EVALUATION FORMS

Evaluative inquiry can be classified conceptually into five categories, or Forms. These have been labeled as follows:

- Proactive;
- Clarificative;
- Interactive;
- Monitoring; and
- Impact.

Below and in Table 3.1, we set out the basic tenets of each evaluation Form by including the following aspects:

- purpose or orientation of an evaluation consistent with the Form;
- typical issues (broad questions) that are consistent with each purpose; and
- major Approaches, taken from a social science or management perspective.

We see the first two of these aspects as fundamental to planning an evaluation that is consistent with the assumptions of that Form.

The third aspect needs an additional comment. It is widely acknowledged in academic circles that social scientists, and in particular those connected with the field of education, have dominated advanced thinking about the work of the evaluator profession. However, there have also been considerable contributions to practice from the management/accounting perspective. That both 'cultures' have something to say about the conduct of evaluation in the workplace is evident to anyone who has attended conferences or meetings of professional associations of evaluators in North America and Europe. Yet, up until now, most evaluation texts have failed to integrate the thinking about evaluation that has emerged from the two cultures. Here we have made an attempt to integrate perspectives where it makes sense to provide a more holistic and inclusive view.

Proactive evaluation

Purpose or orientation

Evaluative inquiry within this Form takes place before a program is designed. Findings assist program planners to make decisions about what type of program is needed. The major purpose is to provide input to decisions about how best to develop a program in advance of the planning stage. Proactive evaluation places the evaluator as an adviser, providing information about the extent of the problem that policy should address, or what program format is needed. Proactive evaluation may provide leaders with 'just in time' advice for making key decisions which affect the future or even survival of an organization.

Typical issues

Issues about which an evaluator might be engaged include the following:

- Is there a need for the program?
- What do we know about the problem that the program will address?
- What is recognized as best practice in this area?
- Have there been other attempts to find solutions to this problem?
- What does the relevant research or conventional wisdom tell us about this problem?
- What could we find out from external sources to rejuvenate an existing policy or program?

Major Approaches

Approaches that are consistent with this Form include:

- *Needs assessment or needs analysis*. This is probably the best-known Approach within this Form, and a strong body of theory and practice has been developed around it. In the past, the evaluation community has perceived needs assessment to be distinct from evaluation, because needs assessment precedes the development of a program. As the name implies, needs assessment involves assessing the perceived community want or need among the community which will be addressed by the projected program.

- *Research synthesis (evidence-based practice)*. This Approach involves a synthesis of what is known about the problem from 'funded knowledge'—in other words, relevant research and other scholarly inquiry. The use of this Approach provides an opportunity for the aggregated work of applied research to impact on social planning and as such represents an attempt to bridge the gap between the work of the research community and applications in real settings.
- *Review of best practice (creation of benchmarks)*. In this Approach, there is an emphasis on selecting and studying exemplary practice which has relevance to the problem that needs to be addressed. The use of the term 'benchmark' has its origins in management, and the trend for businesses in a given field to model their activities on leaders in that field. Similar developments can now be seen in the public sector. It should be noted that the selection and analysis of how exemplary or 'lighthouse' agencies run their businesses is fundamental to the benchmarking activity, but is not the whole story. The creation of benchmarks must be followed by implementation of processes that will deliver more effective and efficient outcomes.

While the 'review of best practice' Approach has been associated with effective private and public sector management, the needs assessment and research review Approaches are more likely to be associated with the work of social scientists. Proactive Evaluation is discussed in greater detail in Chapter 9.

Clarificative evaluation

Purpose or orientation

Evaluative inquiry within this Form concentrates on making explicit the internal structure and functioning of an intervention. This is sometimes described as the theory or logic of a program. The logic of a program attends to the links between program assumptions, program intentions and objectives, and the implementation activities designed to achieve these objectives. The need to outline or define the logic usually arises when a program has not been fully specified or described, even though it is in operation. This can occur when there is pressure for developers to implement an intervention without sufficient opportunity or knowledge to fully develop its rationale, or when those responsible for delivering a program are in conflict over aspects of its design, such as program intentions. Another possibility is that, even though program staff are implementing the program in some way, there is confusion about how the program should ideally be implemented. All these situations call for a *clarificative evaluation*, in which the evaluator usually works with policy or program staff. The *essential element* that distinguishes program planning from Clarificative evaluation is that in the latter, the collection and analysis of data is essential. The involvement of program staff in the development of draft and final versions of the logic is usually encouraged (Rutman 1980; Smith 1989).

Typical issues

Issues about which an evaluator might be engaged include the following:

- What are the intended outcomes of this program and how is the program designed to achieve them?
- What is the underlying rationale for this program?
- What program elements or structures need to be modified to maximize program potential to achieve the intended outcomes?
- Is the program plausible?
- Which aspects of this program are amenable to a subsequent monitoring or impact assessment?

Major Approaches

Approaches that are consistent with this form include:

- *Evaluability assessment (EA).* Evaluability assessment is a well-known technique for developing program logic, and is included here as a separate Approach because of its historical significance. In the 1980s, evaluators developed definitions, examples of practice and guidelines for others undertaking studies of this kind. EA was originally seen as an essential step before further evaluation could be conducted. The aim was to determine if a program could be described in sufficient detail to make it amenable to monitoring or impact evaluation. In other words, the question was whether the program was 'evaluable', hence the rather unusual name.

  While an EA can still be carried out as a precursor to Approaches in other evaluation Forms, it can also stand alone as a means of determining the essential features of a program.
- *Program logic development.* This involves the construction of an explicit description of a program. An essential final product is a

program description portrayed in schematic format, sometimes supported by documentation. A range of schemas can be used, but in most the essential elements are: program assumptions, objectives and implementation activities. Central to program logic is the nature of program causality, the ordering of events in such a way that the presence of one event or action leads to, or causes, a subsequent event or action.

- *Ex-ante evaluation.* An ex-ante evaluation assesses the feasibility and validity of the design of a program. It is designed to determine, at the planning stage, whether a program is likely to be successful in the field, whether it can be implemented as planned, and whether implementation will lead to the stated objectives. Ex-ante evaluations can be thought of as quality assurance checks before extensive resources are committed to the implementation phase. In this Approach the evaluator acts as an independent 'honest broker'. The evaluator may have access to relevant information that program staff may not have—for example, scientific evidence that shows that the intervention will work in the field. Ex-ante evaluation has found particular application in the international development arena in recent times.

Clarification evaluation is the focus of discussion in Chapter 10.

Interactive evaluation

Purpose or orientation

Interactive or participatory evaluation is based on an assumption that those with a direct vested interest in programmatic interventions within organizations or communities should also control the evaluation of these interventions. Representative groups control agendas, and the evaluator (externally or internally based) responds. Interactive evaluations assist with ongoing service provision and structural arrangements, usually with a strong emphasis on process. In some instances, the evaluator may also be involved in facilitating change that is consistent with the evaluation findings (Cousins & Whitmore 1998).

While Impact and Monitoring Forms of evaluation are more likely to provide findings relevant to senior managers and funding agencies, findings provided by evaluations within the Interactive Form are more logically directed at middle level managers and program implementers.

Typical issues

Issues about which an evaluator might be engaged include the following:

- What is this program trying to achieve?
- How is this service progressing?
- Is the delivery working?
- Is it consistent with the program plan?
- How could the delivery be changed so as to make it more effective?
- How could this organization be changed so as to make it more effective?

Major Approaches

Approaches which are consistent with this Form include:

- *Responsive evaluation.* This involves the documentation or illumination of the delivery of a program. In addition to being focused on process, responsive evaluation takes account of the perspectives and values of different stakeholders, and is orientated towards the information requirements of audiences, often the providers of the program.
- *Action research.* This encourages extensive involvement of program providers in the design and implementation of internal evaluations based around the trial of an innovative program, technique or structure.
- *Developmental evaluation.* This involves evaluators working closely with program providers on a continuous improvement process, often on programs that are innovatory and unique.
- *Empowerment evaluation.* This involves assisting program providers and participants in the development and evaluation of their own programs, as part of a broader goal of giving citizens more control over their own lives and their destiny.
- *Quality review.* Sometimes known as 'institutional self-study', this involves providing system-level guidelines within which providers have a large amount of control over the evaluation agenda.

Monitoring evaluation

Purpose or orientation

Typically, monitoring is appropriate when a program is well established and ongoing. The program may be on a single site or it may be delivered at several sites, remote from senior management. Staff are aware of specified goals or intentions, have identified program targets and implementation is taking place. There is usually a need for managers to have an indication of the success or otherwise of the program or one or more of its components. This is likely to be linked to the expenditure of program funds.

An evaluation of this Form may involve the development of a system of regular monitoring of the progress of the program. Typically, *quantitative performance indicators* have been used as the means of organizing data in monitoring evaluations, but more recently we have recognized that data management in any evaluation requires employment of mixed methods. Indicators cannot, in themselves, provide the last word on program effectiveness. Indicator information needs to take contextual factors into account to provide valid and useful findings.

Evaluations within this Form are likely to be driven by a performance management perspective, and key theorists in the area have described the need for evaluation to include a rapid response capability (Mangano 1989) and to provide timely information for organizational leaders (Owen & Lambert 1998).

Typical issues

Issues about which an evaluator might be engaged include the following:

- Is the program reaching the target population?
- Is implementation meeting program benchmarks?
- How is implementation progressing between sites?
- How is implementation progressing now compared to a month ago, or a year ago?
- Are our costs rising or falling?
- How can we fine-tune this program to make it more efficient?
- How can we fine-tune this program to make it more effective?
- Is there a site which needs attention to ensure more effective delivery?

Major Approaches

Approaches which are consistent with this Form include:

- *Component analysis.* This involves the systematic evaluation of a component of a large-scale Program, identified because there are indications that the component needs to be reviewed to bring it into line with organizational goals.
- *Devolved performance assessment.* This involves the development of systems through which component entities can report regularly on their progress.

- *Systems analysis*. This involves setting up procedures by which the central management institutes common evaluation procedures to be used uniformly across a system of agencies or programs.

In all Approaches, the findings provide an indication of performance against some standard, or as a basis for a consequent review (Wholey 1983). Evaluators are likely to be internally located at the center of organizations with access to management information systems (MIS). Alternatively, evaluators might be in the public sector—part of a government department with responsibility for the delivery of a service provided by local agencies, for example, the provision of care of the elderly through nursing homes. In this scenario the department may provide an evaluative structure with which all agencies must comply, and be charged with monitoring the homes. Monitoring evaluation is the focus of discussion in Chapter 12.

Impact evaluation

Purpose or orientation

Impact evaluation is used to assess the effects of a settled program. A logical endpoint for analysis is assumed—for example, establishing the outcomes of a completed adult education remedial reading program or the sustainability of a program of international assistance. Alternatively, an evaluation could be conducted to assess the effects of an ongoing program at a given point in time, such as a mid-term review. An example might be a review of a ten-year housing support program after the first five years of its life.

Typical approaches include the extent and level of attainment of specified objectives, determination of the level of performance on a suite of outcome indicators, or examining both intended and unintended outcomes.

If the intention of the evaluation is to make a decision about the worth of the program (see Chapter 1), evaluations of this Form are described as *summative evaluations*. Summative evaluations assist with decisions about whether to terminate a program or to adopt it in another place. It is important, in many impact evaluations, to determine whether the intervention described in the program plan is in place. Thus, while the emphasis in an impact evaluation is on outcomes, it may also include a review of the implementation characteristics of the program. These studies are known as *process-outcome evaluations*.

Typical issues

Issues about which an evaluator might be engaged include the following:

- Has the program been implemented as planned?
- Have the stated goals of the program been achieved?
- Have the needs of those served by the program been achieved?
- What are the unintended outcomes of the program?
- Does the implementation strategy lead to the intended outcomes?
- How do differences in implementation affect program outcomes?
- Is the program more effective for some participants than for others?
- Has the program been cost-effective?

Major Approaches

Approaches that are consistent with this Form include:

- *Objectives-based evaluation.* This involves judging the worth of a program on the basis of the extent to which its stated objectives have been achieved. It should be noted that objectives-based evaluation represents the foundation of evaluation practice.
- *Needs-based evaluation.* This involves judging the worth of a program on the basis of the extent to which the program meets the needs of the participants. This represents a variation on objectives-based evaluation, and makes the assumption that the objectives of a program do not necessarily represent the needs of the participants.
- *Goal-free evaluation.* This involves determining not only the stated goals, but also the unintended outcomes of the program; thus the common name given to this approach is misleading. Goal-free evaluation has implications for evaluation practice, as looking for unintended outcomes (whether both positive or negative) implies the use of flexible, rather than preordinate designs.
- *Process–outcome studies.* This involves not only determining outcomes but also measuring the degree of implementation of the program. The need for attention to implementation arose from the mistaken notion that social and educational programs were always delivered in ways that were consistent with program intentions.
- *Realistic evaluation.* These studies are based on the principle that it is not possible to ascribe universal or generalizable cause-and-effect statements to any program. Rather, it is only possible to say that a program works under certain conditions. That is, a program is effective in certain circumstances for certain groups of participants in certain contexts.
- *Performance audit.* A performance audit is an analysis of program efficiency and effectiveness. Performance audits concentrate on program outcomes, and generally involve both financial and non-financial measures.

Impact evaluations are often used to justify expenditure, which is consistent with the notion of a summative evaluation role. While such evaluations can be handled internally, external evaluators most often undertake them. Impact evaluation is discussed in detail in Chapter 13.

USE OF FORMS IN FOCUSING AN EVALUATION

It is important for all those responsible for conducting an evaluation to choose the most appropriate way of proceeding. The Forms just discussed provide a conceptual map by which the evaluator and client can make a decision about how to proceed. Example 3.1 illuminates the use of Forms in this way.

Example 3.1 Evaluation of training program for child welfare workers

We were asked to undertake an evaluation of a training program for child welfare workers in a large state agency. In initial negotiations, the stakeholders expressed a strong desire for an impact evaluation based on program goals. After further discussions with the program manager and inspection of program documentation, particularly the course plan and materials provided for participants as handouts, it became evident that the program plan was not specific and that members of the training team were not clear about program themes or how various course components linked together.

These deliberations led to a realization among stakeholders that a Clarificative evaluation was needed. The methodology employed included observation, analysis of all documentation, then some interactive sessions with all members of the training team, including the program manager, to develop a revised program plan.

A key feature of the evaluation was that the training team, through the development process, recognized the need for a more systematic plan, and developed a commitment to implementing a program which had greater internal coherence.

In summary, this was a classic Clarificative evaluation:

- The orientation was towards clarification of course description;
- The program was still in a stage of development;
- The focus of the evaluation was on its design; and
- It was undertaken during cycles of program delivery.

The revised plan became the basis for ongoing delivery of the training program, offered several times. When it was deemed to be settled, the impact evaluation originally suggested by the stakeholders was carried out.

Example 3.1 emphasizes the point that it is essential to take into account the state of the development of a program when deciding on the appropriate evaluation Form (Owen 1991). It would have been illogical to proceed with an outcomes evaluation of an intervention that was incoherent and had little chance, in its original state, of being effective. The evaluative thrust, at least in the first instance, needed to be directed toward program clarification. Later, an outcomes evaluation made sense.

The following scenarios provide an opportunity for you to classify them according to the evaluation Forms just introduced.

Scenario A: The Willand Anti-Violence Project aims to lower the instance of alcohol and drug-related violence across the Willand County. A management team chaired by the head of the local fire brigade oversees the project. The management team has little program design expertise, and, while key members of the team have knowledge of their areas (police, fire-fighting, ambulance, etc), they have few ideas on how to go about implementing the project. A member of the team suggests hiring an expert in violence reduction who also has good people skills. The expert's role includes undertaking small action-research projects in towns in the shire and generally assisting with the development and delivery of the strategy.

Scenario B: Two years ago the Billie Senior Citizens Association initiated a Community Safety Project. The project involves service personnel visiting the homes of elderly people and giving advice about safety. Follow-up visits are designed to check on the implementation of the advice given. The project is well managed by the director of the association, is well designed and 'in place'. The project committee wants a study that will determine whether the project has been effective.

Scenario C: The Ozieland Government has recently instituted a Safe-Towns Program. This involves the development of a policy of improving the general safety levels of people in their day-to-day living. The policy encourages cooperation between town councils and those responsible for safety, and community groups. Initially 27 towns are involved. Senior management wants an indication of how the program is progressing over time.

Scenario D: The Bellet City Board of Management wants to develop a program to reduce the incidence of assault and associated activities in a defined area of the city. A couple of members of the board have strong ideas about what should be done. The chief executive hires a well-known large consultancy firm to develop some options about the nature of the intervention that is needed.

Scenario E: The Scragga City Council had a major street drug problem and obtained a grant to develop strategies to reduce the incidence of drugs on the streets. This involved appointing a program coordinator who was to be responsible for developing an articulated program plan. Some processes have been implemented but, despite the best efforts of the coordinator, an overall program has not been developed. The council wants to produce such a program.

You may decide, for example, that Scenario C can be classified within the Monitoring Form and Scenario E belongs to the Clarificative Form. The importance of this exercise is that we are providing some order in what could be a bewildering array of possibilities for attacking the realities of evaluation practice. There is more guidance at hand to help classify evaluation scenarios and this is provided in the following section.

FORMS OF EVALUATION: ADDITIONAL DIMENSIONS

Table 3.1 provides a summary of the three dimensions we have used to introduce the Forms: orientation, typical issues and key approaches. It should be useful in helping you decide which Form (or Forms) is the most appropriate for a given evaluation situation. However, there are additional dimensions for this conceptual framework. These are described below and outlined in Table 3.2.

- *State* of the existing program. State means the degree to which the program under review has been implemented at the time of the proposed evaluation. State can vary: at one extreme the program will not be in existence and needs to be developed, while at the other extreme, the program will have been operating for

Table 3.1 Evaluation Forms: orientation, typical issues and key approaches

	Proactive	Clarificative	Interactive	Monitoring	Impact
Orientation	Synthesis	Clarification	Improvement	Checking/refining/ accountability	Learning/accountability
Typical issues	• Is there a need for the program? • What do we know about this problem that the program will address? • What is recognized as best practice in this area? • Have there been other attempts to find solutions to this problem? • What does the relevant research or conventional wisdom tell us about this problem? • What do we know about the problem that the program will address? • What could we find out from external sources to rejuvenate an existing policy or program?	• What are the intended outcomes and how is the program designed to achieve them? • What is the underlying rationale for this program? • What program elements need to be modified in order to maximize the intended outcomes? • Is the program plausible? • Which aspects of this program are amenable to a subsequent monitoring or impact assessment?	• What is this program trying to achieve? • How is this service going? • Is the delivery working? • Is delivery consistent with the program plan? • How could delivery be changed to make it more effective? • How could this organization be changed so as to make it more effective?	• Is the program reaching the target population? • Is implementation meeting program benchmarks? • How is implementation going between sites? • How is implementation now compared with a month ago? • Are our costs rising or falling? • How can we fine-tune the program to make it more efficient? • How can we fine-tune the program to make it more effective? • Is there a program site which needs attention to ensure more effective delivery?	• Has the program been implemented as planned? • Have the stated goals of the program been achieved? • Have the needs of those served by the program been achieved? • What are the unintended outcomes? • Does the implementation strategy lead to intended outcomes? • How do differences in implementation affect program outcomes? • Is the program more effective for some participants than for others? • Has the program been cost-effective?
Key Approaches	• Needs assessment • Research synthesis (evidence-based practice) • Review of best practice (Benchmarking)	• Evaluability assessment • Logic development • Ex-ante	• Responsive • Action research • Developmental • Empowerment • Quality review	• Component analysis • Devolved performance assessment • Systems analysis	• Objectives-based • Needs-based • Goal-free • Process-outcome • Realistic • Performance audit

Table 3.2 Evaluation Forms: all dimensions

	Proactive	Clarificative	Interactive	Monitoring	Impact
Orientation	Synthesis	Clarification	Improvement	Checking/refining/accountability	Learning/accountability
Typical issues	(see Table 3.1)	(see Table 3.1)	(see Table 3.1)	(see Table 3.1)	(see Table 3.1)
State of Program	None	Development	Development	Settled	Settled
Major focus	Program context	All elements	Delivery	Delivery/outcomes	Delivery/outcomes
Timing (vis-à-vis program delivery)	Before	During	Mainly during but could be at other times	During	After
Key Approaches	• Needs assessment • Research synthesis (evidence-based practice) • Review of best practice (Benchmarking)	• Evaluability assessment • Logic development • Ex-ante	• Responsive • Action research • Developmental • Empowerment • Quality review	• Component analysis • Devolved performance assessment • Systems analysis	• Objectives-based • Needs-based • Goal-free • Process-outcome • Realistic • Performance audit
Assembly of evidence	Review of documents and data bases, site visits and other interactive methods. Focus groups, nominal groups and delphi technique useful for needs assessments.	Generally relies on combination of document analysis, interview and observation. Findings include program plan and implications for organization. Can lead to improved morale.	Relies on intensive onsite studies, including observation. Degree of data structure depends on approach. May involve providers and program participants.	Systems approach requires availability of management information systems (MIS), the use of indicators and the meaningful use of performance information.	Traditionally required use of pre-ordinate research designs, where possible the use of treatment and control groups, and the use of tests and other quantitative data. Studies of implementation generally require observational data. Determining all the outcomes requires use of more exploratory methods and the use of qualitative evidence.

a period of time without modification. If a program can be described in this way we refer to it as being fully implemented or 'settled'.

- *Focus* of the evaluation. Focus refers to the program component(s) on which the evaluation is likely to be concentrated. For a given program four possible foci are:
  - the social, political and economic context in which a program is to be developed;
  - the coherence and adequacy of program design;
  - elements of program delivery or implementation; and
  - program outcomes.
- *Timing* refers to the temporal links between the evaluation and program delivery. For example, evaluations consistent with the Proactive Form take place before a program is developed, while those consistent with Monitoring evaluation occur over time as the program is being delivered.
- *Assembly of evidence*. This refers to the methodology and techniques selected: the design of the empirical part of the evaluation process. In evaluation studies, the questions drive the selection of *data-management techniques*. Data management involves things such as sampling, choice and application of data collection techniques and analysis. The end point is to arrive at findings that address the evaluation questions.

In summary, each Form can be classified by the seven dimensions represented in Tables 3.1 and 3.2. The inclusion of the variables 'state of program', 'focus' and 'timing' imply that different forms of evaluative inquiry are related to different stages of program development. That is, a Proactive evaluation would logically precede the development of a given program, and an Impact evaluation can be thought of as an evaluation that takes place at the conclusion of a program.

USING THE FORMS IN PRACTICAL SETTINGS

The Forms should be regarded as conceptual or heuristic devices that aid planning of real evaluations. They are designed to act as a guide to thinking about evaluative inquiry and the different meanings we have given it. It is now time to apply these ideas to practical situations. How can we make these ideas operational to guide evaluators, clients, audiences and other interested parties through the conduct of a given evaluative study? Consider the following example.

Example 3.2 Using a combination of Forms to plan a large scale evaluation: The National Evaluation of the Supported Accommodation Assistance Scheme (SAAP)

SAAP is a combined Commonwealth and states program designed to fund and administer services to the homeless in Australia. Since it was established about 20 years ago, it has become the major policy focus for providing assistance to homeless people across the country. Over 1200 agencies provide services and in 2003 over 140,000 clients were given assistance. SAAP policy is evaluated every five years as a major input into future policy development relating to homelessness.

In 2003, an evaluation of the fourth cycle of the program (SAAP IV) was undertaken by Erebus Consultants. After extensive consultations with the key stakeholders, the following evaluation issues were developed to focus the evaluation:

- *Program effectiveness*. What outcomes have been generated? How had they have been achieved to meet the needs of diverse clients?
- *Program accountability*. Has compliance worked? Has the program's management (at national and at jurisdictional levels) worked? Has expenditure been tracked? How have stakeholders seen program accountability?
- *Program efficiency*. How much was spent for what outcomes? What is the cost of homelessness to society generally? Has there been improvement both administratively and at service levels relative to previous performance levels?, and
- *Future directions*. What should constitute policy to address homelessness in the future? Are there alternative ways of implementation that would be more effective? Is there policy divergence or convergence between stakeholders? (Wyatt et al. 2004).

The Erebus team produced the following framework in Figure 3.1 as the basis of designing the evaluation, from which we can see that the evaluation was conceived in terms of two of the evaluation Forms. The first was Impact, which concentrated on effectiveness, accountability and efficiency; the first three of the issues listed above. The second was Proactive, and sought to provide information drawn from the context. The Proactive component related in particular to the fourth and last of the issues listed above. This is a good example of linking evaluation issues to Forms, and provided conceptual clarity for the evaluation team. Note that the Figure 3.1 also lists the methodologies used in the evaluation design of the Proactive component—for example, summaries of emerging research, best practice, etc.

Figure 3.1 Combined use of Proactive and Impact Forms in an evaluation

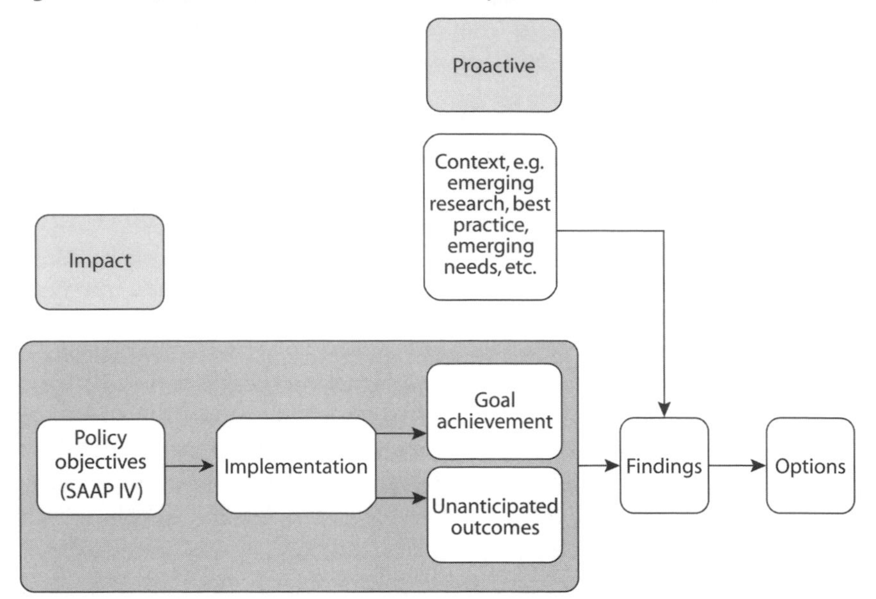

Adapted from *National Evaluation of the Supported Accommodation Assistance Program (SAAP IV) Final Report*, 1994. Erebus Consulting Partners, May 2004.

Evaluation forms and change management

Faye Lambert has linked Evaluation Forms to business and management principles (Lambert 1996). This work is grounded in the change management literature and the work of Kotter (1995) in particular. Based on observations from about 100 organizations, Kotter suggests that eight critical steps are required to successfully manage a major organizational change initiative. They are:

1 *Building a case for change*. Key stakeholders, such as staff and shareholders, need to understand why change is necessary, thus the evidence supporting the change must be collected and articulated to those affected by it. Change is about risk, so the risk of not changing needs to be perceived as greater than the risk of going ahead with it.
2 *Forming a powerful guiding coalition*. This involves molding a group of individuals into an effective team and providing them with enough power to lead the change effort.
3 *Creating the vision*. What is initially required is a sense of direction, not myriad plans. There is a need for those involved in the change

effort to share the vision, which could come from a charismatic leader or be developed by a coalition.

4 *Communicating the vision.* The nature of the vision needs to be communicated synergistically to stakeholders.
5 *Empowering others to act on the vision.* This requires administrators to set up structures to support the change and to remove potential obstacles standing in the way of its introduction.
6 *Planning for and creating short-term wins.* This is about ensuring tangible signs of improvement early on in the initiative to provide momentum for furtherance of the change. In association with this, there should be opportunities to recognize and celebrate success.
7 *Consolidating improvements.* This involves incorporating the change into the very fabric of the organization. This almost always involves both person-centered and resource support from the administration.
8 *Institutionalizing new approaches.* This involves making sure that those within the organization make the connections between the change and outcomes which follow from the change. This is done with a view to ensuring that the coalition understands and supports the change.

These steps are set out in Figure 3.2. While the diagram implies a linear sequence, the truth is that implementing change is far more messy, with plenty of recursive loops involving the steps set out above.

Where does evaluative inquiry fit into this change scheme? Critical diagnostic evaluation should be an integral part of decision-making related to the change process. Lambert's research suggests that the average manager spends about 80 percent of the available time on implementation, with only around two percent spent on diagnosis, whereas she suggests that 20 percent of management time should be spent on the diagnostic effort, and just 40 percent on implementation. We suggest that a major reason for this discrepancy is that, up to now, the typical manager has had limited understandings of how diagnostic evaluation can aid the change effort.

We show how these links can be forged in Figure 3.3. Proactive evaluation would be employed in Steps 1 and 2. Clarificative evaluation would be employed in Steps 3 to 6, and so on.

Imagine that a small, forward-looking university has made an in-principle decision to introduce information technology across all departments. The administration decides to use evaluation to help in introducing an information technology policy. A Proactive evaluation could be based around the following questions:

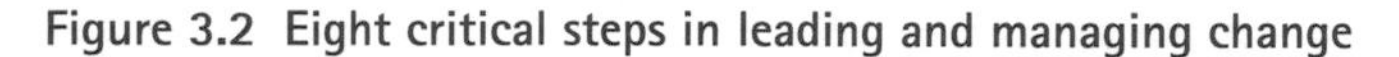

Figure 3.2 Eight critical steps in leading and managing change

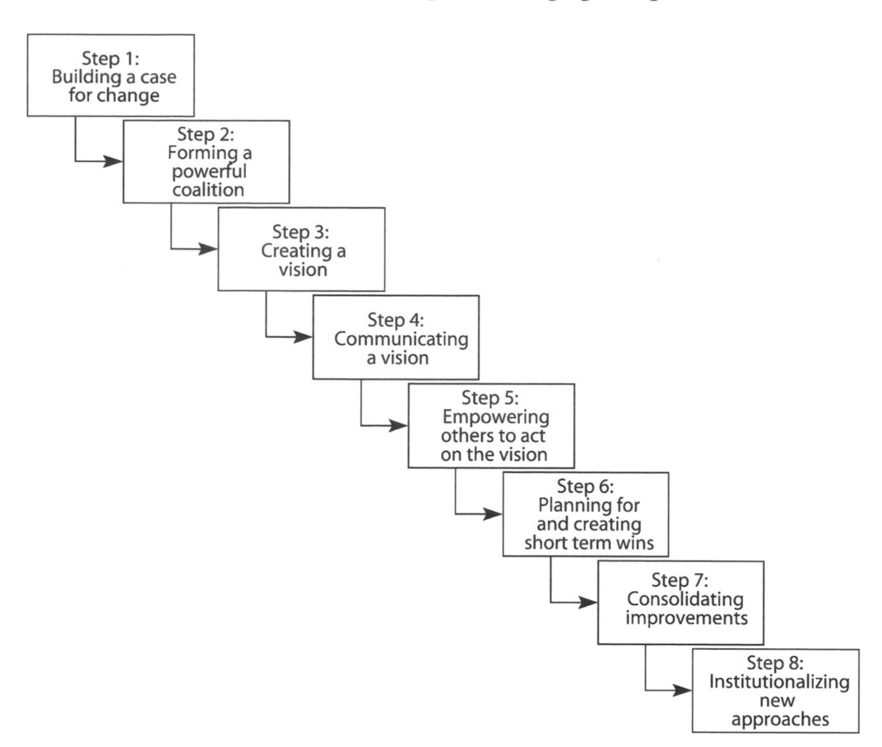

Figure 3.3 The change process and the use of evaluative inquiry

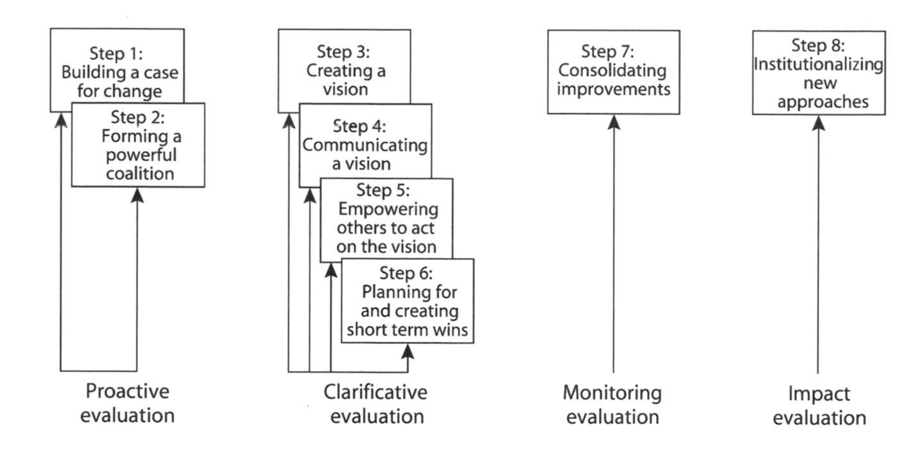

- What are the skills and abilities that will enable students to effectively participate in and shape their world of the future?
- What do we know already about the potential of information technology to help meet their needs?

- How might technology be used to develop those abilities in this university context?

To get people onside, a case for the change must be made, particularly among those with clout, those who Kotter describes as the 'powerful coalition'. Proactive evaluation would involve engaging staff in discussions about how they could use technology, not simply to familiarize students with technology, but how to use it proactively in reshaping the 'college curriculum'. Actively involving the coalition in leading staff through a needs analysis would be one way of building support for the change effort.

A Clarificative evaluation would be undertaken in conjunction with Steps 3 to 6 of Figure 3.3: the design and development of the information technology policy. Typical questions would be:

- What are the intended outcomes from the implementation of the policy?
- What are the underlying assumptions?
- What would it mean to the work of each department if the policy were implemented?
- What aspects of the program should be chosen for Monitoring or for Impact evaluation?

The evaluative effort to this stage has resulted in:

- development of a clear understanding of the intended outcomes of the policy and the strategies used to achieve them;
- a basis for monitoring evaluation process for the program in action; and
- a basis for future modifications, because the original policy has been based on explicit identification of policy need.

Similar questions could be developed for the Monitoring evaluation phases (see Figure 3.3).

Experience suggests that if staff are involved, there is increased understanding that most worthwhile innovations take time to implement. The use of evaluation not only provides useful knowledge, but also helps clarify expectations for the different stages of policy development. Clarifying expectations goes hand in hand with clarifying policy. This alleviates much of the anxiety of the change initiative and can assist with ongoing policy implementation.

Perhaps the most important message from these examples is that 'real evaluations' can span one or more of the evaluation Forms. The following is another example of this.

Example 3.3 Evaluating the progress of a skills management program

Maher (1996) employed several evaluation Forms in relation to an innovative teaching program designed to assist students at risk of dropping out of high school. The program was of one week's duration and was held before the beginning of the conventional school year. Program content focused on research skills, task and time management, and report writing. The study reflected the use of several Forms and Approaches which were consciously used in conjunction with the program over a fifteen-month period. They included:

- needs analysis prior to and in the early stages of planning;
- monitoring during the program;
- needs-based outcomes evaluation, designed to answer the question 'Was it worth doing?', to account for the use of resources, to identify the effects on students, and to document what was done (Maher 1996).

CONCLUSION: AN EPISTEMOLOGICAL BASIS FOR THE FORMS

Evaluation Forms provide an overarching framework to assist those involved in planning an evaluation. The introduction of Forms is a manifestation of the move from evaluation as the judgment of worth, to evaluation as the production of responsive empirical knowledge. The fact that there are five Forms suggests that evaluation should no longer be seen as a unitary concept. Rather, it implies that there are five dominant styles of evaluation, and that each of them produces useful knowledge for decision-making. This extends the reach and influence of evaluation well beyond that of solely determining the worth of a program.

Table 3.3 summarizes this position and is organized around two concepts: Assumption and Imperative. *Assumption* provides an epistemological basis for carrying out evaluative work within this Form. So, for example, the Proactive Form is based on an assumption that what is already known about a given problem—and which could be ameliorated through a programmatic intervention—should be brought to bear on the design of that intervention.

Imperative amplifies the notion of Purpose to include the importance of the Form, a fundamental characteristic, which, presumably would be acceptable to stakeholders who commission that Form of evaluation. For example, in the Proactive Form, a commitment to

Table 3.3 Epistemological bases of Forms

Form	*Proactive*	*Clarificative*	*Interactive*	*Monitoring*	*Impact*
Purpose	Synthesis	Clarification	Improvement	Checking/ refining/ accountability	Learning/ accountability
Assumption	What is already known should influence action	Program rationale and design needs to be laid out	Those close to action need information for ongoing change	Programs need to be monitored to ensure quality	Need to know what works and why
Imperative	Importance of external frame of reference	Importance of making intervention explicit	Importance of provider involvement	Importance of quality control	Importance of transferability: contribution to funded knowledge

using external relevant information in designing the program would be important to the stakeholders.

Taken together, Assumption and Imperative can be thought of as representing a value position regarding the role of evaluation and, by implication, what knowledge is important. While Forms can be used to complement each other in a given evaluation, it is also possible that evaluators and stakeholders exhibit a preference for one Form over another. There is for example an inherent tension between the Interactive and Monitoring Forms and their use in an organization. While one encourages the use of democratic principles in the determination of what needs to be evaluated, the other takes a management control position, supporting the right of managers to use evaluation resources for their own agendas.

These issues will be explored in more depth later in this book. To encourage the intelligent use of each of the Forms we go into more detail about each one in Chapters 9 to 13. Conceptually, this involves working down the columns of Tables 3.1, 3.2 and 3.3.

REFERENCES

Cousins, J. B. and Whitmore, E. (1998). Framing participatory evaluation. *New Directions for Evaluation*, 80, Winter 1998, 5–23.

Day, S. (1991). *Casework Evaluation*. Unpublished Paper for the Graduate Diploma in Evaluation, Centre for Program Evaluation, The University of Melbourne.

Kotter, J. P. (1995). Leading change. Why transformation effects fail. *Harvard Business Review*, March–April 1995, 59–67.

Lambert, F. C. (1996). *The Introduction of Technology into Classrooms: Change Management and the Role of Evaluation*. Paper presented at the Expanding Horizons Conference, Geelong College, Geelong, Australia.

Maher, M. (1996). *Educational Evaluation*. Unpublished Major Project for Doctorate of Education, Faculty of Education, The University of Melbourne.

Mangano, M. F. (1989). *Rapid Response Evaluation for Decision Makers: The Story of the HHS Inspector General*. Washington DC: US Department of Health and Human Services.

Owen, J. M. (1991). An Evaluation Approach to Training Using the Notion of Form: An Australian Example. *Evaluation Practice*, 12(2), 131–139.

Owen, J. M. and Lambert, F. C. (1998). Evaluation and the Information Needs of Organizational Leaders. *American Journal of Evaluation*, 19(3), 355–365.

Patton, M. F. (1996). A World Larger than Formative and Summative Evaluation. *Evaluation Practice*, 17(2), 131–144.

Rutman, L. (1980). *Planning Useful Evaluations*. Beverly Hills: Sage.

Shadish, W., Cook, T.D. and Leviton, L.C. (1991). *Foundations of Program Evaluation*. Newbury Park: Sage.

Smith, M. F. (1989). *Evaluability Assessment: A Practical Approach*. Norwell, MA: Kluwer.

Stufflebeam, D. S. and Webster, W. L. (1983). An Analysis of Alternative Approaches to Evaluation. In G. F. Madaus, M. Scriven & D. L. Stufflebeam (eds), *Evaluation Models*. Boston, MA: Kluwer-Nijhoff Publishing.

Wholey, J. (1983). *Evaluation and Effective Public Management*. Boston: Little, Brown.

Wyatt, T., Carbines, R., Willett, J., and Robb, L. (2004). *National Evaluation of the Supported Accommodation Assistance Program (SAAP IV)*. Canberra: Commonwealth of Australia.

4 Negotiation and Evaluation Planning

In Chapter 1 we adopted a description of evaluative inquiry as the processes of:

- developing an evaluation plan;
- implementing an evaluation design to produce findings;
- disseminating findings to identified audiences.

All three stages are essential to the practice of evaluation. Their execution requires evaluators to possess a range of complementary skills. In the first stage, the emphasis is on *planning*. Interpersonal skills are required in dealing with stakeholders: those who have a legitimate interest in the program. In the second stage, the emphasis is on *data management*: the collection and analysis of evidence. This is sometimes referred to as the *obtaining stage*. Methodological skills are required. In the third stage, the emphasis is on *information dissemination strategies* and *reporting*. Communication skills are required.

While for conceptual purposes we imply that the stages, as outlined, follow each other, in practice they might overlap. For example, in an evaluation in which one phase of data management is dependent on the findings of a prior phase, the evaluation could be conducted as a set of rolling stages of planning, obtaining and disseminating. It should also be noted that the stages are interdependent. For instance, planning is designed to establish the scope of the evaluation and thus set the parameters for the obtaining stage.

The need to develop planning and communication skills in addition to data management skills cannot be over-emphasized. Good evaluation is more than the ability to gather and manipulate evidence. This applies whether the evaluator is an outsider, working for an agency that undertakes evaluation work on contract, or an insider, working for the organization which has commissioned the evaluation.

The inclusion of the planning and communicating stages helps to distinguish evaluation from some other social science research. While both evaluation and research draw on a similar range of data collection and analysis techniques, the conduct of research and evaluation have different epistemological characteristics:

1 Compared with research, evaluators must devote considerable energy and resources to ensuring that an adequate and acceptable plan is developed, and that evaluation findings are comprehensible to clients. In an evaluation of college level programs for training teachers, it was estimated that 30 percent of the resources available for the study were devoted to the planning and dissemination stages of the study (Owen et al. 1985), leaving 70 percent for the obtaining stage. It is important for evaluators to budget for planning and communicating in addition to obtaining when allocating available resources for an evaluation.
2 Research is concerned with general explanations designed to advance the frontiers in a discipline or field of study. A major motivation for research is the search for generalizations and the creation of new concepts and theoretical perspectives. By contrast, evaluation concentrates on specific policy or programmatic interventions and is motivated by the need to inform decisions about those interventions (Smith & Glass 1987).
3 Those undertaking research are answerable to the scientific community at large, while evaluations are commissioned inquires. Evaluators are beholden to some or all of the stakeholders.
4 Most scholars undertaking research attempt to take a disinterested value position, while an evaluator could have an interest in the program, and adopt a 'critical friend' position as a means of influencing the use of the findings.
5 While there is often a high commitment to elaborate designs and flexible time-frames in the conduct of research, evaluators must adopt a pragmatic perspective, often selecting from a limited range of evidence from which to present findings, make conclusions, and meet deadlines. This applies in particular to *post hoc* evaluations, that is, evaluations occurring after the program has commenced or completed.

Now that we have a firmer view about the meaning of evaluation in practice, we turn to a description of each of the major stages of evaluative inquiry. In the remainder of this chapter we examine the planning stage. The obtaining or assembly of evidence stage is examined in Chapter 5, and the dissemination stage is discussed in Chapter 6.

Before we examine planning in detail, we wish to discuss briefly the related issue of negotiation in evaluation.

NEGOTIATING IN EVALUATION

Effective planning and dissemination requires the development of effective negotiation skills on the part of the evaluator. Fundamental to the ideal of negotiation is the concept that evaluators perform a service to clients who require answers to specific questions about a given program or policy. Evaluators must be prepared to acknowledge the interest framework of the client, and ensure that the knowledge they produce has salience to ensuing decisions about the evaluand under review.

Up to now most professional evaluators have felt their way in negotiation. Evaluators have worked with stakeholders in the conduct of evaluations without the benefit of knowledge of effective negotiation techniques. Markiewicz (2005) suggests that a theory of negotiation should be based on both the mediation and social conflict literature, and the evaluation literature. Some results of her research are summarized below.

The mediation and conflict literature asserts that the effective negotiator needs to have highly developed skills in both empathy and assertiveness, and the ability to discern when to lean toward one attribute rather than the other. The negotiator thus needs to be conversant, skilled, and sensitized to both the affective and instrumental aspects of the negotiation context. The negotiator thus operates in a domain which balances task-oriented problem-solving with due attention to process, atmosphere, use of language, enhancement of self-awareness and awareness of the variety of positions being promoted.

Thus, negotiation may be viewed as facilitating a consciousness-raising process, whereby the parties become aware of each other's positions, and of the rationale underpinning these positions. Through this process, there is a journey towards enlightenment, which facilitates a shared process of problem-solving. Problem-solving is a by-product of the enhanced understandings achieved, a transformative process, rather than a focus in and of itself. Negotiations progress through certain stages and phases, which, when recognized, can assist in managing the process. In the initial stage in negotiation positions are taken and put on the table, the middle stage is where there is active negotiation, and the last stage is where steps are taken to reach consensus.

From the perspective of a practicing evaluator, Owen (1998) identified three key considerations in developing a theory of negotiation within evaluation. These are 'the identification of key players; determination of what is negotiable and when negotiation should take place; and the establishment of the reasons for negotiation, why it is important' (pp. 33–35). By 'key players' we mean those stakeholders who have a voice in the negotiation process. These are the program stakeholders who, for one reason or another, are consulted by the evaluator during the evaluation. Key players can be the representatives of stakeholders on the evaluation reference or steering committee. A key player could also be someone not formally represented on a steering committee but who, for one reason or another, is consulted about the conduct of an evaluation.

From the above there emerges broad scope for negotiation during *all* stages of the evaluation process, from inception to finalization.

Conflict and differences in perspectives among key players/ stakeholders, and between key players/stakeholders and the evaluator, can emerge at any time. It is consequently important for the evaluator to be in a position to respond to these differences in both a timely and competent manner, so that further stages in the evaluation process are not impaired by unresolved conflict.

Stake (1983), Patton (1997) and Fetterman et al. (1996) all recognize conflict as inherent in the evaluation process. They see the evaluator as a consciousness-raising agent who should expect value differences among evaluation clients, and create an environment conducive to reconciling them. Guba and Lincoln (1989) assert that the evaluator should be a facilitator in the negotiation process, with the goal of arriving at understanding as opposed to consensus.

More recently, Owen (1998) identifies the following four areas about which negotiation can take place within an evaluative activity:

1 Overarching principles of the evaluation:
   - orientation or purpose of the evaluation;
   - models or Approaches to be taken into consideration;
   - value set for making judgments.
2 Key player/stakeholder involvement within the evaluation and the role of the evaluator:
   - respective roles and responsibilities of stakeholders and the evaluator in operationalizing the evaluation.
3 Details of design and methodology:
   - the evaluation design and data management processes to be employed;
   - key questions or issues to be answered.
4 Recommendations, findings and utilization:
   - nature of the conclusions, judgments or recommendations to be made;
   - identification of who will be involved in the creation of knowledge products and action associated with the findings.

NEGOTIATION AND EVALUATION PLANNING

A major milestone that needs to be reached through negotiation is an evaluation plan. While there may be differences in emphasis in the degree of planning, effective use of evaluation findings is heavily dependent, in all arrangements and settings, on the degree to which evaluator and clients agree on a plan for the evaluation. This is the up-front agreement that determines the directions the evaluation will then take.

Attention must be given to client involvement in the planning stage of an evaluation, *before* any data collection or analysis takes place. There must be reasonable agreement between evaluator and client about the broad parameters of the evaluation so that the parties are clear as to how it will proceed, and are aware of what the evaluation might realistically be expected to achieve.

Negotiation is fundamental because it sets the direction of what follows—it determines what questions are important, and to whom they are important. Negotiation helps in other ways. Clients can be advised that some questions cannot be answered, due to the fact that the evidence is not available—for example, because baseline data had not been gathered. In addition, the evaluator should outline ways in which information about the evaluation and the findings of the evaluation will be disseminated. Up-front planning through negotiation builds in support for the evaluation effort.

As outlined in the previous section, there is often a diversity of views among stakeholders about the purpose of an evaluation. Different interest groups associated with a given program often have different agendas, and it is essential for the evaluator to be aware of these groups and know of their agendas from the beginning. One solution to this situation is to determine the questions that are of interest to each of these groups and to devise data techniques that produce findings for each of these questions. If this is the evaluation design adopted for an impact evaluation, it follows that program worth becomes relative rather than absolute (see the discussion in Chapter 1). That is, a program could be judged to be worthy from the criterion questions of one interest group but not from those put forward by another group.

Such a design is difficult to manage. An alternative is to ensure that all interest groups can be represented on a committee that manages the evaluation. It is then the task of the committee to develop an agreed set of questions as a basis for discussions with the evaluator.

In practice we find that many evaluation committees are made up of one or two stakeholder groups. They are usually also the clients or audiences for the findings, and it is with these groups that the evaluator negotiates about the evaluation design; elements such as the key issues to be addressed, the timeline and budget (see later for an elaboration of these elements). This does not mean that the findings or products of the evaluation are necessarily restricted to these audiences. Other stakeholders may also receive these findings or products. However, the evaluation design may not answer questions that these stakeholders would like to ask about the given program, nor will the styles of reporting be specifically tailored to their wishes or needs.

An evaluation plan should be settled in advance of other evaluative actions. The plan could be regarded as an agreement between the evaluators and the client(s) about the direction the evaluation will take. This does not mean that everything that follows is set in stone, to be followed in an unyielding fashion. For example, there might be agreement that the direction of the evaluation is determined by what has been found in a previous round of inquiry and reported back to the primary audience. However, it does mean that the general direction of the evaluation has been decided, and that this direction will be followed unless circumstances are such that follow-through is impossible—for example, if the expected data sources are unavailable. In this case, the evaluation plan should be renegotiated.

A FRAMEWORK FOR PLANNING AN EVALUATION

While evaluation plans can have a variety of formats, we have found that the following headings provide a logical and helpful way of presenting the plan.

Specifying the evaluand

What is the object of the evaluation? What is known about the evaluand? How was it developed? How long has it been in existence? What is the nature of the evaluand: policy/program/organization/service? Who are the key players in its development (actual or projected) and its implementation?

Purpose

In terms of the Forms presented in the previous chapter, what is the fundamental reason for commissioning the evaluation? As we have seen, the fundamental purpose of a given evaluation might be to prove that a given intervention is effective, to improve the delivery of an intervention, or to help develop an intervention. We have discussed the primacy of the evaluation Form in determining the orientation of different kinds of evaluative inquiry. This implies that a plan for a Proactive evaluation would look very different to a plan for Monitoring evaluation. Consistent with evaluation Form, a key issue is whether the evaluation is primarily concerned with:

- synthesis of information to aid program development;
- clarification of a program;
- improvement of the implementation of a program;
- monitoring program outcomes; or
- determining program impact.

Clients/audiences

To whom will the findings of the evaluation be directed? As indicated above, it is important to distinguish between the clients, the primary audience for an evaluation and other interested parties. The primary audience is the individual or group that is most likely to use the knowledge, in the form of evidence, conclusions, judgments or recommendations. Note that the primary audience is not necessarily identical to the commissioners of an evaluation, defined as the group that initiates and provides the resources for the evaluation. The identification of the primary audience(s) implies that it is difficult for a given evaluation to provide the information needs of a wide range of stakeholders. Patton (1997) found that the identification of an influential individual during the course of an evaluation can significantly affect the utilization of evaluation findings. We agree. However, on the basis of working cooperatively with organizational members, we have also found that there is often a key small group within an organization for whom the evaluation has particular meaning, and who can encourage an ongoing commitment to using evaluation findings (Owen 2003). Thus an individual or a small group of individuals may have influence over decisions relating to the program under review, and their involvement is vital during the negotiation stage of the evaluation.

Resources

What person power and material resources are available to undertake the evaluation? Someone must be given time to plan, to set up appropriate data management systems and generally to be responsible for all aspects of the evaluative inquiry. External evaluators develop structures for coping with the realities of running what is often a complex operation. However, more and more, government departments and not-for-profit agencies have developed internal arrangements so that evaluations can be undertaken in-house—for example, departments which have separate budgets and other resources, and trained staff to make evaluation work feasible across an organization (Love 1994).

We believe that resources must be identified and made available, even in the case of small-scale studies in which there may be no clear distinction between evaluation and development/implementation tasks—for example, in the Action Research Approach. If program deliverers are also expected to engage in evaluation, they should be given time and resources to undertake their research within the range of other day-to-day tasks. The inclusion of this element reminds us that evaluations are always done under resource and time constraints; in fact, the resources available determine the extent of the data management and the range of evaluation findings that can be provided to the primary audiences.

Focus

What is the nature of the object or evaluand under review—for example, is it a policy or program or organizational unit? Which elements or components are to be reviewed—for example, the program plan or its implementation? What is the state of development of the evaluand?

The identification of the focus ensures that the evaluators are clear about the object to be investigated, so that the highest quality information can be produced given the resources available.

Evaluation issues and key questions

This involves the selection of the most important aspects of a program to be examined. In practice, this is the way in which an evaluation can be made more manageable because it forces clients to think about the fundamental directions the evaluation will take.

It is quite common for an evaluation management committee such as a school council or a group of middle-level managers to put forward a long list of issues they would like addressed. The evaluator may need to work with the client to reduce this list. This involves educating the client about the realities of working within a budget, challenging them as to the relative importance of each issue, and identifying those questions that are not amenable to answers through the evaluation.

For the purposes of planning, issues should be turned into a set of evaluation issues as broad questions. These questions serve to focus the evaluation even more and provide a direction for the collection and analysis of data. Posing a small set of key questions is fundamental for the evaluation to go forward. The nature of key questions is discussed in more detail in Chapter 5.

Assembly of evidence/data management

For each issue a collection and analysis strategy should be developed. It is important that the data-collection and analysis techniques chosen should be those that best answer the questions. The implication is that the evaluator should have recourse to a repertoire of data-collection and analytical strategies, and an understanding that, in the end, there is a need for the evaluator to make sense of the evidence and draw defensible conclusions. The range of data management techniques possible is wide, and it is in this area that a trained evaluator or someone with research skills is often needed.

Dissemination of findings

How will information about the evaluation be disseminated? How will the findings and conclusions arising from the evaluation be disseminated? Is there a need for recommendations? If so, who will create them?

It is a truism that many evaluations have not had an impact on decision-making because the evaluator has not used effective techniques for disseminating the findings. In particular, the long and esoteric report has been shown to be ineffective in transferring information. More creative techniques are called for, including those that allow clients and evaluators to interact. Also, when making decisions about reporting, the evaluator should bear in mind the sophistication of the audiences and, if possible, ensure that findings from the analyses can be presented in ways that make sense to them. It is fundamental that clients comprehend the findings of the evaluation and understand their implications. The issue of whether recommendations will be developed by the evaluators or by others should be considered during the planning phase of the evaluation. Dissemination is discussed in more detail in Chapter 6.

Codes of behavior

What are the ethical conditions which underlie the evaluation effort? Standards of conduct underlie the work of professionals such as doctors and psychologists. Evaluators should also ensure that high ethical standards are applied to the conduct of an evaluation. These are discussed in detail in Chapter 8.

Budget and timeline

Some indication of the amount of resources needed for the evaluation should be included in the evaluation plan. If an evaluation is to be carried out externally, it is necessary for the evaluators to cost their services and associated resources, and to set them out clearly. Working out a week-by-week work schedule helps ensure that the evaluation will be well managed and that the findings will be delivered on time. A schedule must take into account the resources that are available for the investigation. It is important that resources and time are allocated to the negotiation and dissemination phases of the evaluation.

While it is advisable that the evaluation plan be set out under a set of discrete headings, we wish to emphasize that the overall plan should be coherent—that is, the entry under one heading should be consistent with those under *all* other headings. There is no use planning an elaborate data collection effort related to many evaluation questions if the budget is $500! In practice, getting to a final evaluation plan generally involves a series of steps. The first one is to respond to the information provided in an evaluation brief, or to the broad concerns of the clients if a formal brief is not available. Generally, the initial brief provides the basis for a second step, discussions between client and evaluator, which leads to the third step, a final evaluation plan.

This refinement is the part of evaluation negotiation without which there is a high likelihood that the remainder of the evaluation effort will be unsatisfactory to all parties. These processes may take up to 15 percent of the total evaluation budget.

An issue is whether an external evaluator should withdraw if they find that there is some aspect of the proposed evaluation, or the program, with which they have some moral or ethical concern. It should be made clear that the negotiation can include these concerns, and that the final evaluation plan should take into account suggestions from the evaluator in addition to addressing the perceived needs of the evaluation commissioners.

In the course of an ongoing evaluation, it may be necessary to develop a series of evaluation plans as the needs of the client(s) change over time. It is not necessary for an entire plan to be finalized prior to the first round of data collection. It is possible for an evaluation to have a series of phases, each dependent on one that has gone before. For example, in a study we conducted some years ago, the evaluation team worked to provide feedback on the trials of an innovatory curriculum designed to increase the participation of girls in school mathematics and science courses. Over a period of a year, the evaluation team negotiated a series of mini-plans which directed data collection on selected trials. Each of these phases lasted about six weeks. A mini-plan for a subsequent period was to some extent dependent on what had been found in the previous six weeks. This was an example of a situation where the evaluators provided a highly responsive service to program developers. It should be emphasized, however, that for all phases a mini-plan was negotiated to the satisfaction of the evaluators and the program team.

An evaluation planner suitable for use in negotiating evaluation is included as Figure 4.1.

Figure 4.1 Negotiating evaluations: dimensions of an evaluation plan

1. **Specifying the evaluand**
   What is the focus of the evaluation?
2. **Orientation or purpose(s) of the evaluation**
   Why is the evaluation being done?
3. **Clients/primary audiences**
   Who will receive and use the information?
4. **Evaluation resources**
   What person power and materials are available?
5. **Evaluation focus/foci**
   Which element(s) of the program will need to be investigated: program context, program design, program implementation, program outcomes or a combination?
6. **Key evaluation issues/questions**

- *Assembly of evidence/data management*
  What are the key questions and how can we collect and analyze data to answer them?
  For each question, outline the data management techniques to be used.
- *Key questions*
  To what extent does ... ?
  Is there ... ?
  In what ways does ... ?

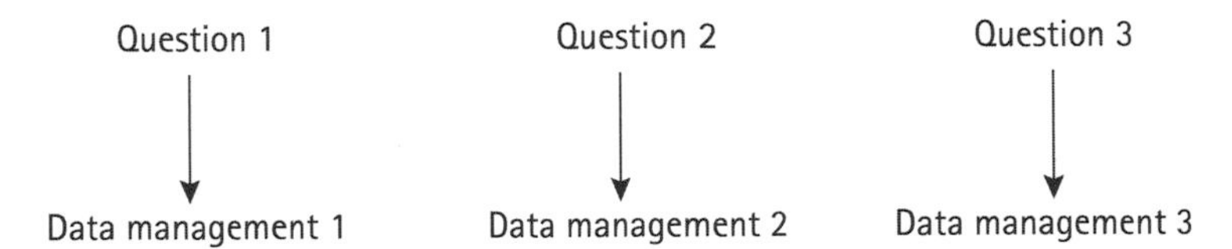

Figure 4.1 (*continued*)

- ***Data management***
  What are the most appropriate methods of data collection and data reduction?
  Collection (some considerations)
  - Is sampling important?
  - Is anything known about this from other sources?
  - How will the data be collected?

  Analysis and interpretation
  - How will the data be analyzed to address the key evaluation question?

7 **Dissemination**
- What strategies for reporting will be used?
- When will reporting take place?
- What kinds of information will be included (findings, conclusions, judgments, recommendations)?

8 **Codes of behavior**
What ethical issues need to be addressed?

9 **Budget and timeline**
Given the resources, what will be achieved at key time-points during the evaluation?

10 **Other considerations that emerge in the course of the negotiation**

THE IMPORTANCE OF EVALUATION PLANNING

If a plan is not negotiated, an unsatisfactory evaluation in practice is likely to be the outcome, as the following example shows.

Example 4.1 Evaluation of a national school improvement program

This example concerns a national evaluation of school improvement, the Participation and Equity Program (PEP). The first stage of the evaluation was specifically devoted to the development of an evaluation plan. The plan proposed that the evaluation consist of several phases with differing methodologies. For example, one phase involved an analysis of the reaction of different systems (state education departments and private school systems) to PEP. A second phase involved a set of case studies in school and community colleges.

While the plan paid extensive detail to methods, it lacked specificity on other elements of an evaluation plan. For example, there was insufficient attention given to the purposes of each phase, the major audience for the phase, and the likely uses of the findings. There was a general agreement among the evaluators that the national commissioning agency needed to know about PEP, but beyond this there was a lack of clarity about the reasons for the evaluation.

One result was that each phase was carried out as if it was a research study with minimal interaction between clients and evaluators. There was also little interaction between staff working on each phase. As each phase was completed, reports were forwarded to the commissioning agency.

A question which arose among those responsible for the case studies was: Why are these being undertaken and for whom? The best guess was that they were primarily aimed at enlightening bureaucrats about the impact of their policies at the grassroots level. This was an acceptable use of the case study evaluation findings, but was never made specific at any stage during the design or implementation of the evaluation. If it had been negotiated, the case study evaluation team may have decided on more effective forms of reporting other than those used: a series of case reports. For example, an alternative with more likelihood of enlightening key bureaucrats could have been a seminar at which the site developers described their programs and the evaluators followed with a critical review of these programs.

As it was, a decision was made to publish and distribute the case studies to school and school systems twelve months after they had been forwarded to the commissioning agency. Presumably they were seen as being of primary value to practitioners, not to bureaucrats.

If the evaluators and commissioners had decided that practitioners were to be the primary audience, this almost certainly would have had an impact on how the case studies were planned and how the findings were disseminated.

In summary, the evaluators should have devoted more attention during the planning stage to the social interactive elements and less time to data management. They needed to arrange things so that the evaluation messages were more timely—to set up arrangements through which the bureaucrats could request information when it was needed. It would also have been useful for those concerned if there had been some face-to-face meeting between clients and evaluators through the year. These aspects should have been part of the evaluation design but were not brought up during the initial planning stage of the project.

AN EVALUATION PLAN: AN EXAMPLE

Recently, a large city (BigTown) commissioned an evaluation plan with an external evaluator, with a view to moving on to the data management stage of the study. The focus of the study was the SafeT Program, an attempt by BigTown City Council to improve the quality of life across the metropolis. A meeting was held between the commissioner of the study, the Director of Social Programs at BigTown, and the evaluator. At this meeting the evaluator also had recourse to key documents about the SafeT Program. Subsequently the following evaluation plan was prepared.

Example 4.2 Evaluation plan for the SafeT Program

Introduction

This document provides an evaluation plan for the SafeT Program (hereafter, the STP), a major program currently being undertaken by the BigTown City Council and a number of partners.

The evaluation plan should be regarded as indicative, a basis from which those working directly on the STP and the Council can make decisions on the final orientation of the evaluative approaches to be used.

This strategy is based on the notion that those most closely associated with the Program, the key stakeholders, need to be involved in final decision-making in order to build commitment to the evaluation processes and the utilization of the evaluation findings.

These procedures are designed to ensure that key stakeholders have a common understanding, up front, of what the evaluation hopes to achieve, and the products it will deliver.

Based on the negotiation, a final design for the study should be agreed so that the study can proceed to the data management phase.

Structure of the evaluation plan

For this discussion, the tentative plan is established under a set of headings which, taken together, represent an integrated evaluation design. The headings are as follows:

- Object of the study
- Orientation of the evaluation
- Audiences for the evaluation
- Key questions

- Data management
- Reporting
- Timeline and resource implications.

Setting out the proposal for the evaluation under these headings is predicated on an assumption that there are links between them. That is, the plan should be coherent across headings rather than each being seen as independent. This form of planning:

- assists in identifying the key issues to be explored;
- identifies the audience(s);
- ensures that the evidence and conclusions address the key issues of the identified audiences; and
- encourages the utilization of findings.

So while each area must be treated in turn, it is essential that the reader understand that links must be drawn across the areas.

Object of the study

In discussing an evaluation design, it is also important to identify clearly the object which is the focus of the evaluation. By object of the study we mean the 'thing' being evaluated. An object can be a policy, a program, a product or a combination of these.

Understanding the nature of the object, its intentions, implementation and planned outcomes, makes subsequent discussions of the evaluation purposes clearer. This, in turn, assists in the development and implementation of the data management phase of the study—that is, decisions about what data to collect and how to analyze it.

For the purposes of clarity, we make the following distinctions between 'objects':

- *Policy* expresses intentions about directions in a given organization that have priority. The Policy in a given area gives guiding assumptions and goals for that area.
- *Programs [capital P]* are administrative umbrellas for distributing and regulating funds under a policy. Experience suggests that while there are one-off Programs, many government programs have extended lives and directions which are only changeable at the margins.
- Programs consist of *projects*, the actual delivery of specific interventions. Projects may differ widely in character: while some are permanent, others may have lives which are shorter than those of the Program of which they are a part. In

addition, there can be variation in the location of projects and in the personnel involved. Sometimes, projects are referred to as '*little p*' programs.

In this case a major object under consideration is the STP, that reflects the BigTown City Council's policy on safety for citizens. The strategy and the STP are based on the following policy directives:

- a broad and cooperative approach to city safety;
- safe streets and neighborhoods;
- safe transport;
- well-planned and appropriate controls;
- activities and special events that are safe for all; and
- a reduction in criminal and anti-social behavior.

In keeping with the generic distinctions above, current STP projects include:

- revitalization of the west precinct of the city;
- establishment of an accord with proprietors of licensed bars and clubs;
- installation of public surveillance systems in selected areas; and
- training for Council's staff in community safety principles.

The object about which conclusions and decisions need to be made is the STP Program. In order to make these decisions and conclusions, the objects which will be the focus of attention are:

- the documentation and implementation of the STP. This includes ways in which the Program responds 'up' to Council policy, and 'down' to the delivery of specific projects; and
- the documentation and delivery of specific projects. This includes the degree to which the projects are consistent with the intentions of the STP, and the individual impact of these projects.

Orientation of the evaluation

Orientation refers to the primary purpose and how the evaluation will be conducted to meet the knowledge needs of the audience(s).

The orientation suggested here implies the use of an external evaluator who will work closely with the primary audience: key Program staff. This is based on the notion that the STP is an ongoing program, and that key staff need to have access to evaluative information on a continuous basis in order to:

- make modifications, from time to time, to the Program's objectives and administration;
- make decisions about the effectiveness of existing individual projects, including whether they should be extended, modified or terminated;
- make decisions about the introduction of new projects under the Program;
- keep key decision-making bodies, such as the SafeT Executive Committee and the BigTown City Council, informed of the progress of the STP. They, in turn, need to decide at a given point whether the Program should be terminated, or amalgamated with other Council initiatives.

This is consistent with what we term *Monitoring evaluation*. A key element is that the evaluator is seen as an essential support for program leaders. Evaluators involved must have a range of evaluation skills; they must also possess knowledge of program planning, and must have the ability to respond rapidly and flexibly to the needs of key audiences. A feature of the work of the evaluator is to provide relevant high-level information to staff for decision-making. This role can be contrasted with a more intensive evaluation in which the emphasis is on large-scale 'end-of-program' evaluation designed to 'prove' that the program has been a success.

The approach to evaluation suggested here is one in which the evaluator adopts a stand consistent with an interested but unbiased expert. It should be stressed that the evaluator would *not* be involved in any aspects of program delivery. Thus an element of 'distance' is maintained between the evaluative and delivery functions.

Clients/audiences

The reason for identifying key audiences is to ensure from the outset of the data collection and analysis that the issues for investigation and the dissemination strategies are the most appropriate for them.

From what has gone before, the primary audience for the evaluation is the program management of the STP. We would expect the evaluator to report to the primary audience in a variety of ways, some of which may be informal, and will involve direct interaction with key Program staff. An important issue is the provision of relevant and timely information about those aspects of the Program which have high priority at a given point in time.

There are, of course other audiences for the findings of the study. We regard the secondary audience to be members of the BigTown City Council.

The secondary audiences may wish to make decisions, at *specified points* in time, about the worth of the STP—say, eighteen months after the evaluation commences. One way for this to be facilitated is for the evaluator to provide an aggregation of information collected throughout the life of the Program. It should be recalled that these data will be used for *ongoing* decision-making by the STP staff. We see this as a second important reporting strategy to be undertaken by the external evaluator.

The use of aggregated data in this way allows the evaluator to effectively address the information needs of both primary and secondary audiences. This is a key aspect of this evaluation design.

Key questions

The following questions could be asked at any point in time in the delivery of the STP. In keeping with an evaluation for management approach, an issue for the evaluator is to provide evidence on the existing situation, and to encourage management to consider how the Program could be fine-tuned to lead to improvement.

Program level

- To what extent is the STP consistent with international best practice? How could the Program be modified to be more in line with best practice?
- To what extent is the STP affecting the general level of safety in the city? How could the Program be modified to be more effective?
- To what extent are the objectives of the STP reflected in the design and implementation of individual STP projects? How could consistency between Program and projects be increased?
- How effective has the administrative decision-making of the STP been in terms of making links between policy and practice? How could the Program be modified to be more in line with community needs?

Project level

For an individual project:

- Is the project plan consistent with the STP?

- What is actually happening within this project?
- Is it meeting the objectives of this project?
- Should it be continued?

Note that these questions apply to each individual project. Posing questions of this nature implies *following a given project over time*. This would be consistent with the needs of the Council to undertake a longitudinal study into the effectiveness of the STP. The number of projects to be followed will be limited by the resources available for the evaluation. Selection of the projects to be monitored should be guided by the priorities of the primary and secondary audiences.

Data management
Data management is the term used to assemble evidence from which evaluation questions such as those above can be answered. It should be noted that there is no one 'formula' for obtaining relevant information for a given question. This implies that the evaluator selected for the work must have a range of skills, including those of collecting and analyzing data for the evaluation questions.

It is our view that:

- an evaluation at Program level is essential;
- the selection of projects to be evaluated would be negotiated, depending on priorities and resources available for the evaluation.

Program level
The following is indicative of how the evaluation questions related to the Program could be handled. For simplicity, we have concentrated on the 'what is' (as distinct from the 'how could the situation be improved?' element) for each question here.

- To what extent is the STP consistent with international best practice?
  Review of literature on benchmarking; elite discussions with selected respondents to identify best practice sites; telephone interviews with managers of identified sites; development of criteria for best practice; review of STP in terms of these criteria.
- To what extent is the STP affecting the general level of safety in the city?
  Development of indicators that reflect the objectives of the Program and their operations; selection of procedures by

which data on these indicators could be collected systematically at given time intervals. Note that this will require some creative attention to data management, as most available indicators may have limited face validity.

- To what extent are the objectives of the STP reflected in the design and implementation of individual STP projects? How could consistency between Program and projects be increased?
  Evaluator review of STP documentation; review of decision-making processes associated with selected projects; review of project documentation and interviews with project leaders.
- How effective has the decision-making of the STP been in making links between policy and practice?
  Individual interviews with key stakeholders, such as senior administrators; use of expert panel on policy implementation.

Project level

One common test that can be applied to projects is to determine whether they are consistent with the objectives of the Program. The evaluators should provide the STP with a method for this checking process.

However, as there will be a wide variety of projects, each one having its own objectives, evaluation of the implementation and outcomes of individual projects will require its own methodological approach.

It is likely that resources will not allow all projects to be evaluated for outcomes. The evaluator should work with the STP to set priorities in this regard.

Dissemination

There should be a high degree of interaction between the evaluators and client audiences for the study. This view is based on research that shows that there is an increased probability of evaluation findings being used if there is a strong link between the evaluators and stakeholders during all stages of an evaluation project.

As indicated above, there are two distinct major audiences for the findings of this evaluation:

- The primary audience is the management of the STP. It is proposed that the evaluator use a range of approaches for reporting to the management. Consistent with the need for timely reporting, it is envisaged that the evaluator will prepare a series of short reports on selected aspects of the STP and its component projects.

- The secondary audience are the BigTown City Council members. It is envisaged that the evaluator will assist the STP management to prepare overview reports summarizing the overall impact of the project at determined points in time. This could be at the end of each year of a three-year project.

Timeline and resource implications

Finally, while a detailed budget for this study has not been developed, there are implications for the amount of funding which would be needed. One is that new Programs need time for implementation, and that implementation is essential for outcomes to be achieved. Most major interventions need at least two years to 'bite'; the more complex the program the longer is the period needed. The second, implied in this plan, is that evaluators should be 'on tap' regularly during implementation to provide quality information as the Program proceeds.

We believe that the study should be undertaken over a 27-month period, beginning immediately. The wishes of the Council to gauge the impact of the study over an extended period are thus consistent with what we know from other studies about the need to evaluate over a period, thus allowing the effects of a program to emerge.

EVALUATION PLANNING AND THE INFLUENCE OF EVALUATION FORMS

While it is interesting to examine an evaluation plan developed by others, as in the example above, there is no substitute for doing a plan yourself. If this is not possible, you might like to develop a tentative plan for the following scenario.

Example 4.3 Developing an evaluation plan

Chapelton Community Health Centre (CCHC) offers a two-day educational program designed for 15–16-year-olds currently attending school.

The program was devised to meet a perceived need for accurate information about issues such as pregnancy, contraception, sexually transmitted diseases and the impact of drugs on the development of fetuses and young children. It is delivered by a team consisting of two CCHC nurses and a visiting gynecologist.

The Program was originally offered to students from nearby schools but as it has become more widely known, most school groups travel to the CCHC by bus. All groups are accompanied by a teacher.

The Centre's manager has provided support for the program through the provision of facilities and nurses' time, but the major mission of the CCHC is to support the general health needs of the local inner urban community.

The Program has two parts. The first involves sessions being taught by the team in a formal teaching–learning situation. Some use is made of videos, slides and charts.

In the second half of the Program, students visit a hospital where additional sessions are held and visits are made to laboratories and wards.

*The Program has been running for several years and is settled as far as the delivery staff are concerned. However, they are finding it difficult to cope with the increasing number of school requests. For the first time, CCHC has an interest in documenting the impact of the Program with a view to having it adopted at other sites. The State Department of Health and Well-being has made a grant of $15,000 to fund the study. It is the beginning of a new year. You are a member of a small external evaluation agency that has been approached to evaluate the program. You have been asked to attend a meeting at the agency before meeting the clients. Use the evaluation planner to develop a tentative plan for the study.

Note that in this case you have been asked to 'scope' the evaluation plan before the negotiation actually begins. We would like to reiterate, at this point, that interaction with the client is essential to finalizing the plan before proceeding to data collection and analysis.

Now, just imagine that all the parameters in the example were kept constant except that which is preceded by an asterisk. Let's change this to the following:

* The Program has been running for almost a year. While the deliverers believe that the Program is generally OK, they need access to information designed to refine it. It is the beginning of a new year. You, as a member of the CCHC with some evaluation experience, are asked to convene a working party and undertake an internal evaluation. In all, there is the equivalent of one person's time for six weeks to carry out the study, and $2,000 for expenses. A plan is needed as the basis for undertaking the evaluation.

You might like to repeat the planning exercise and make a comparison of your two plans.

You will have now realized that the evaluation plan and subsequent stages of the evaluation would be very different for the two scenarios presented in Example 4.3. The first calls for an impact study focused on outcomes and thus is consistent with the Impact Form. The second calls for an internally based improvement-focused study concerned with program delivery, and is consistent with the Interactive Form.

CONCLUSION

As Barrington (1990) has noted, college training programs have tended to focus on evaluation designs and methodologies while neglecting skills needed to undertake the negotiation and dissemination stages of evaluation practice. This has left many neophyte evaluators ill-equipped to cope with the pressures encountered in the real world of organizational decision-making and policy evaluation. We believe that the guidelines presented in this chapter will assist evaluators develop more effective negotiation and planning strategies which are essential to sound evaluation practice.

REFERENCES

Barrington, G. V. (1990). *Evaluation Skills Nobody Taught Me, or What's a Nice Girl Doing in a Place Like This?* Paper presented at the Annual Meeting of the American Evaluation Association, Washington, DC.

Fetterman, D. M., Kaftarian, S. J. and Wandersman, A. (1996). *Empowerment Evaluation: Knowledge and Tools for Self-Assessment and Accountability*. Thousand Oaks, CA: Sage.

Guba, E. G. and Lincoln, Y. S. (1989). The countenance of fourth generation evaluation. In D. J. Palumbo (ed.), *The Politics of Program Evaluation*. Thousand Oaks, CA: Sage.

Love, A. (1994). *Internal Evaluation: Building Organizations From Within*. Paper presented at the International Conference of the Australasian Evaluation Society, Canberra.

Markiewicz, A. (2005). A balancing act: Resolving multiple stakeholder interests in program evaluation. *Evaluation Journal of Australasia*, 4, (1/2), 13–21.

Owen, J. M. (1998). Towards a theory of negotiation in evaluation. *Evaluation News and Comment*, 7(2), 32–35.

Owen, J. M. (2003). Evaluation culture: A definition and analysis of its development within organizations. *Evaluation Journal of Australasia*, 3(1), 43–47.

Owen, J. M., Johnson, N. J. and Welsh, R. J. (1985). *Primary Concerns: A Project on Mathematics and Science in Primary Teacher Education.*

Melbourne, Vic: Melbourne College of Advanced Education, for the Commonwealth Tertiary Education Commission.

Patton, M. Q. (1997). *Utilization Focused Evaluation.* 3rd ed. Thousand Oaks, CA: Sage.

Smith, M. L. and Glass, G. V. (1987). *Research and Evaluation in Education and the Social Sciences*. Englewood Cliffs: Prentice-Hall.

Stake, R. A. (1983). Stakeholder influence in the evaluation of cities-in-schools. *New Directions for Program Evaluation*, 17, 15–30.

From Evaluation Questions to Evaluation Findings

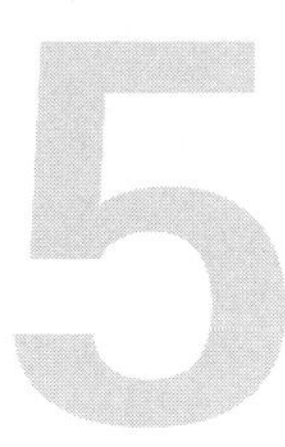

In this chapter we link the negotiation/planning stage of the evaluation process to the obtaining or empirical stage. This includes consideration of the evaluation design—managing data or evidence through the use of relevant methods or techniques. It may not be a surprise to learn that social scientists, philosophers and others have engaged for some time in discussions about the nature of evidence and, more broadly, the underlying bases of inquiry on which research about social phenomena is based. It is useful to outline some of these issues briefly before turning to their relevance for evaluation practice.

PARADIGMS OF INQUIRY IN EVALUATION

At the basis of these discussions is the notion of an *inquiry paradigm*. This is:

> a set of interlocking philosophical assumptions and stances about knowledge, our social world, our ability to know that world, and our reasons for knowing it, assumptions that collectively warrant certain methods, certain knowledge claims, and certain actions on those claims. A paradigm frames and guides a particular orientation to social inquiry, including what questions to ask, what methods to use, what knowledge claims to strive for, and what defines high quality work (Greene & Caracelli 1997, p. 6).

A philosophical position about inquiry has implications for the selection of sources, and for the gathering and making sense of data. In recent times, two major paradigms have become pre-eminent. These are:

- *Post-positivist.* Based on a view that social phenomena not only exist in the real world, but that systematic and stable relations exist between them. The regularities that link phenomena together can be expressed in terms of lawful or causal relations or constructs that underlie individual and social life. The aim of inquiry is to prove or discover lawful or causal relations between elements of the phenomena. Studies consistent with this paradigm seek to establish generalizable knowledge. The fact that most of these constructs are neither tangible nor visible does not make them invalid. Traditionally, proof-focused studies have used large-scale data sets and relied heavily on quantitative methods. Discovery-focused studies tend to be smaller in scale and have relied more heavily on qualitative methods.
- *Constructivist.* Based on a belief that reality, or at least social reality, is socially constructed—that is, there is no objective reality. The aim is not to find the 'right' description of a program, but to develop an increasingly sophisticated description that incorporates multiple perspectives. An evaluation based on this paradigm would focus on gathering constructions, descriptions and analyses from relevant people, including intended clients, staff and others, jointly reflecting on them, and seeking synthesis and consensus. Evidence would be useful to fill out these descriptions but would not 'prove' their validity. Typically, studies within this paradigm are inductive in nature, adopt an investigatory perspective, and provide knowledge that is specific to the context. There is an emphasis on intensive study, often concentrating on a small number of cases or sites, and on the use of quantitative methods.

An issue that has been occupying the minds of evaluation theorists is the degree to which these 'world views' and others have, and should, impinge on the practice of evaluation, and in particular the use of different methodologies. A consensus is now emerging that, while we should be aware of the paradigms mentioned above, evaluators could or should adopt an alternative perspective that is known as:

- *Emergent realism.* Like the post-positivist perspective, this paradigm assumes the existence of an external reality. It assumes that social researchers and evaluators, by the use of a combination of systematic methods, can provide an accurate perspective of this reality. The more adequately we select and apply these methods, the closer we will get to an accurate description or rendering of this reality. However, a key aspect of the emergent realism perspective is that we must always be aware of the tentativeness of our findings. Emergent realism holds that a synthesis of evidence from the use of appropriate methods is needed to provide a rich and adequate understanding of programs and their effects (Henry et al. 1998).

The emergent realism paradigm implies methodological *pragmatism*. According to Datta (1997), an evaluation design needs to be practical, contextually responsive and consequential, so we should ask:

- Can salient questions be adequately answered?
- Can the design be successfully carried out?
- Is there an optimization of trade-offs in the use of different methods—for example, between breadth and depth of understanding of an issue related to a given question?
- Are the results usable?

These are key points for evaluation practice as outlined in this book. We take the view that salient issues and questions are the drivers of the data management phase of evaluation practice. *The choice of methodological techniques follows from the questions asked, not vice versa.* This is a challenge for social scientists, particularly those who come to evaluation practice with a preference for one methodology over another. Employing an investigator with a limited range of data management skills can lead to the evaluation being methodology dominated, rather than directed by the negotiated concerns of stakeholders.

So in developing an evaluation design, ensuring that the data management strategy will provide robust answers to the key questions is essential. The remainder of this chapter is thus devoted to:

- issue and question development; and
- evaluation design: ways in which these questions can be answered through empirical inquiry.

THE NATURE OF EVALUATION QUESTIONS

The primacy of evaluation issues and questions (hereafter questions) in evaluation has been long been recognized. For example, one theorist says that 'clarification of and discrimination between the various types of questions which evaluations undertake to answer is absolutely fundamental to getting a useful answer at all' (Scriven 1980, p. 46). One way of drawing attention to relevant evaluation questions is to locate them within the five evaluation Forms.

To understand how different styles of questions can be linked to different Forms, we make use of a case study in the area of adult literacy and basic education (ALBE). The project was comprehensive in scope and funded by a national education agency. Initially, practitioners working on ALBE policy were surveyed to determine:

- ways in which the goals of programs they presented were developed and implemented;
- use of procedures that demonstrated the success or otherwise of programs;
- evaluation instruments used; and
- the general level of expertise in evaluation in the adult literacy and basic education community.

Subsequently, it was decided that adult literacy and basic education would be enhanced if guidelines were prepared which made evaluation more meaningful at all levels of ALBE provision. It was also decided that evaluation should not be undertaken in isolation from a larger frame of reference that took into account program design and delivery.

A framework designed to encourage effective evaluation planning was prepared by Lambert and colleagues (1995). Subsequent to this, an extensive professional development program was implemented, based on the framework. A key element of the framework was to assist in setting evaluation questions. Tables 5.1 to 5.5 are derived from those developed for the ALBE framework.

Table 5.1 contains typical *generic* questions that would structure studies consistent with the Proactive Form. An important feature is the inclusion of levels of provision:

- Policy development
- Big P program provision
- Little p program provision.

These could be seen as equivalent to the mega, macro and micro levels discussed in Chapter 2.

Tables 5.1 to 5.5 are in the same format, providing a smorgasbord of generic questions that could be asked by stakeholders and audiences relating to a given initiative. It is important to note that in a given evaluation, those negotiating the evaluation would need to decide on *specific* questions relating to a given policy or program.

Table 5.1 Proactive evaluation: typical questions

Evaluation undertaken to make decisions about a given impending intervention.

	Typical questions	Focus	Clients
Policy level (taken at the national level)	What are the current national agendas, priorities, contexts and goals? What part can ALBE play in achieving national goals? Why do we need a Program and what should be its goals? What are the current literacy skills of the population? Are there specific areas of need? Which should receive priority? How should resources be allocated to service the total range of needs identified?	Current situation and contexts, policy and goals Existing infrastructure, skill levels, present and future needs.	Congressional committees. federal departments and agencies
Big P Program level (taken at the regional level)	What are the particular needs of this region? What are the region's policies, objectives and priorities? Do they address these needs and are they consistent with national policies, objectives and priorities? What is already happening to meet the region's needs? What else would make the difference? Where should we see new provision or innovative provision?	Current situation, contexts, policies and goals Existing Program provision, infrastructure, present and future needs	Funding agencies, regional planning groups
Little p program level (taken at the provider level, e.g. community college/group within community college)	Are our program policies, objectives and priorities consistent with regional, state and national policies, objectives and priorities? Do they provide a framework for the program? What is the present and future need for the program? Do we know who and where our potential program users/students are? How does our program relate to other programs in the area? What are the local conditions that may impact on our program now and in the future?	Current situation, context, program policy and objectives Existing program design, present and future needs	Funding agencies, policy makers, program planners and deliverers

Table 5.2 Clarificative evaluation: typical questions

Evaluation undertaken to make explicit the essential features of a given intervention.

	Typical questions	Focus	Clients
Policy level (taken at the national level)	What are the objectives of our policies? Do our policies have internal coherence? Do our policies provide support for program implementation at the regional level? Are our policies plausible in terms of guidance for practice? How does the national infrastructure support program implementation in line with policies? Do resource allocation practices reflect our stated objectives and priorities? Does our manpower planning adequately support program development?	Policy statements Program information and support	Congressional committees. federal departments and agencies
Big P Program level (taken at the regional level)	What are the objectives of our Programs? Do our Programs have internal coherence? Are our Programs plausible in terms of guidance for practice? Is the rationale for offering each Program clear to all involved? Is it clear as to how we will disseminate Programs? Do providers know what is expected of them in terms of reporting back? Are Program resource allocations transparent from the provider perspective? Are the principles and objectives of staff development Programs designed to support implementation well-developed?	Program statements. Program information and support	Regional staff/ advisory groups, providers
Little p program level (taken at the provider level, e.g. community college/group within community college)	Are our programs consistent with regional objectives? Are they realistic? How are our programs structured to achieve these objectives? Are our program plans internally consistent? Has the program logic of our programs been validated? Which of the present programs should be targeted for an impact evaluation?	Program design Program design	Program planners, program staff and college administration

Table 5.3 Interactive evaluation: typical questions

Evaluation undertaken to make decisions about improvement of a current and/or continuing intervention.

	Typical questions	Focus	Clients
Policy level (taken at the national level)	Are the national strategies designed to address literacy needs working? Are these areas in need of improvement? How effectively is the present infrastructure supporting the needs of the states? Are the personnel management policies appropriate or should there be changes? What are the strengths and weaknesses of the professional development delivery strategies? Are there further areas of professional development which are required to improve state, regional and provider operations? How are policies on resource allocation/distribution and curriculum affecting the states/territories, regions and providers?	Processes	Congressional committees. federal departments and agencies
Big P Program level (taken at the regional level)	How are present Programs affecting providers? Are changes required in priorities for individual Programs? What difference is the funding making to the quality of Program delivery in the region? How can we improve the delivery of the Program? How can we improve the support for the Program?	Processes	Regional authorities/ funding bodies
Little p program level (taken at the provider level, e.g. community college/group within community college)	What actually happens in this program? What are practitioners doing that is working well? What is not working so well? How are students affected by the program in action? Is the delivery tailored to meet individual needs and goals of students? Are professional development strategies, as identified by staff, effective? How has professional development affected program implementation? How could we generally improve the program for the future?	Processes	Program managers/ program staff and clients

Table 5.4 Monitoring evaluation: typical questions

Evaluation undertaken to provide checks on the state of a current continuing intervention.

	Typical questions	Focus	Clients
Policy level (taken at the national level)	How many people are participating in the programs? Are literacy skills increasing? What is the effect of Commonwealth expenditure for this policy area; can this policy be administered more efficiently? Is the money allocated to strategic areas being expended efficiently? What is the cost of identified outcomes? What difference is increased funding making to the type of student outcomes? How much are we spending on each student? Are our policy guidelines clear and well understood? Are they influencing program provision? Do we need to improve our information dissemination?	Existing policy and related program	Congressional committees. federal departments and agencies
Big P Program level (taken at the regional level)	How well are our Programs going? Are they understood by providers? Are they being translated into practice? How many students are graduating from each Program? How does this compare with the situation last year? Has there been an impact on the achievement of student learning outcomes and, if so, how does it compare with last year? Are there differences in achievement at different Program sites: if so, why? How are our regional support mechanisms working; are they as good as last year? Are there differences in the quality of support across the region? What effect is this having on the quality of Programs offered in the region?	Existing Program and related Programs	State and regional authorities funding agencies
Little p program level (taken at the provider level, e.g. community college/group within community college)	How many students are achieving success in our program; how does this compare with last year? What is the attrition rate from our program, compared with other program sites? Are our clients getting jobs or improving job options; is this increasing or decreasing? What proportion of our students are going on to further studies, compared with graduates from similar programs? Does our program exemplify national/regional good practice? Is professional development support acceptable? How much does it cost to run this program?	Existing programs	Managers and program staff, program coordinators and staff

Table 5.5 Impact evaluation: typical questions

Evaluation undertaken to assess the effects of a given intervention.

	Typical questions	Focus	Clients
Policy level (taken at the national level)	How was policy implemented? Were national goals and targets achieved? Was the expenditure justified in terms of gains in literacy and national productivity? Was this the result of the policy initiatives or were other factors involved? Were some regions more successful in implementing their program than others? To what extent was our policy dissemination effective? How well managed was the policy/program interface? Is the policy still appropriate? What should be the direction of future policy in this area?	Existing policy and programs	Congressional committees. federal departments and agencies
Big P Program level (taken at the regional level)	To what extent have regional goals been achieved? Were the real goals reflected in Program statements? Have some Programs performed better than others in achieving desired outcomes? Should some Programs be encouraged over and above others? Have there been any unanticipated outcomes, desirable or undesirable, as a result of the Programs? To what extent were the regional support mechanisms effective in supporting Program provision?	Existing Program	Policy makers and planners, funding bodies
Little p program level (taken at the provider level, e.g. community college/group within community college)	To what extent was our program implemented? Did implementation lead to the stated outcomes? Were there any unanticipated outcomes? What were the short-term and long-term outcomes for our students? To what extent did the program meet the needs of the students? To what extent did regional support affect the implementation and outcomes of the program?	Existing program	Regional staff, program managers and staff

REFLECTING ON THE NATURE OF EVALUATION QUESTIONS

It is clear that there are different styles of questions among the many that have been posed in Tables 5.1 to 5.5.

Difference *is* associated with the Form of evaluation. Different Forms imply different evaluation purposes, so one would expect that questions asked within one Form would be different from those posed within another Form. A factor which contributes to between-Form difference is the *timing* of an evaluation. Let us confine ourselves here to questions asked at the policy level across the five tables. In Table 5.1, Proactive evaluation questions relate to what *ought* to be, to help decision-makers establish a desirable state of affairs. Proactive evaluation is designed to assist with policy development. Ideally, we would like Proactive evaluation to establish that a given intervention is of sufficient quality in terms of solving or ameliorating a given social or educational problem. Compare this with questions asked in the Monitoring Form, Table 5.4. Time has passed, and the policy has been implemented. The policy-maker is now concerned with reviewing what is happening across regions, and maybe at individual sites. There is a concern now with management decisions, those which can assist the policy-maker to 'report up' to senior bureaucrats, and in some cases to fine-tune policy direction. So, at different times, there are different evaluation questions that should be asked.

Within each Form, a factor that influences question style is the *level* of Program provision. Policy-level questions are generally different to Program-level questions. In reality, the evaluation-based concerns of staff differ depending on their needs for information about the intervention under consideration. Consider the implementation of a given policy. While the policy developer may need to know how much the implementation of the policy actually costs, at the site level the program manager's concern could be whether the essential elements for implementation have been assembled successfully. A key question might be whether or not an instructor works well with the students, or whether the teaching or learning facilities are adequate, or the extent to which the students have been briefed as to program expectations.

The *focus* for an evaluation actually changes from level to level. In this example, there is a policy at the national level, at the regional level there is a Program and at the local or provider level there are one or more programs. While there will be differences in these details for other situations, the important distinctions between levels of intervention are likely to remain.

While the style of question asked is linked to Form and level, there are, however, question styles that crop up again and again across all elements in the tables. Perhaps the most pervasive appears as follows: '*What is the situation regarding . . . ?*' or '*To what extent has . . .* ?' or '*What are the . . .* ?' An example of this style from Table 5.1 is 'What are the particular needs of this region?' This is a Program-level Proactive Form question. In Table 5.3 we find the following: 'What actually works in this program?' These questions can be described as *non-causal*—that is, they do not search for cause-and-effect links. The general question style is as follows: 'What is the state of P?' (where P is the intervention—policy, Program or program).

Such a question assumes that we want to know what is happening about P—that is, the assumption is that the evidence in the form of findings and conclusions will be largely in the form of a description of P. If, in fact, P is being delivered at more than one site location, the question implies a cross-site analysis of P to provide comparisons of what is happening within P between sites.

Example 5.1 Evaluation of the Curriculum and Standards Framework (CSF)

The Curriculum and Standards Framework (CSF) was a policy developed by the Board of Studies for use by all schools across a State education system. In addition to general policy, the Board provided schools with curriculum outlines to guide practice. The Board commissioned an external evaluation during the first year of provision.

Among the questions about which senior executives wanted evidence were the following:

- How well is the CSF being disseminated?
- In what ways are schools using the CSF?
- Do the schools value the CSF?

The evaluators collected data by observation, interview and document analysis in a sample of schools over a period of about fifteen months. Findings were presented in the form of charts and tables that summarized patterns across the schools. The primary audience was provided with trend data on dissemination and use at intervals over the fifteen-month period (Owen et al 1996).

Another kind of common question that might be asked is a causal one, along the lines of: What is it in P that causes outcome (O)?

Such a question implies identifying those key elements of P, sometimes called *independent variables*, and their relative contribution to the outcome, sometimes called the *dependent variable*. A study of this nature requires the evaluator to look for evidence within a site or sites that will support the causal links.

The implication of such a question is that the evaluator may need to be involved in the discovery of causal links. This is consistent with an inductive approach to knowledge creation, and is often linked to the use of investigatory data collection and analysis (Miles & Huberman 1994).

Example 5.2 Evaluation of the Curriculum and Standards Framework (CSF)

In addition to the questions outlined in Example 5.1, other questions posed during the CSF evaluation were as follows:

- What is the uptake of the CSF in schools?
- What internal school factors affect the uptake of the CSF?

The second question involved an in-depth analysis of the school-level use of the CSF and a review of factors which seemed to influence use. A 'thick description' of participating schools was prepared. Arising from the case reports, a construct labeled as 'school culture' was identified as a major determining variable—that is, in schools where the uptake was high, school culture was high, whereas in schools where school culture was absent or less evident, uptake was low (Meyer 1997).

It may be necessary to ask whether more of some key variable (or variables) causes more of O? This implies identifying key elements of the Program—let us call them X1 and X2—and their relevant impact on the outcome. To test this, we must have cases where there is variation in the amount of X1 and X2 in the Program.

An evaluation question that encourages this style of inquiry would be as follows: Do different programs of organizational support have differential effects on staff morale? The implications for setting up such a study are that different strategies would have to be implemented, and information collected on their implementation and on changes in staff morale. This is a form of investigation which lends itself to an 'experiment', or the use of *multivariate analysis*, which enables the relative effects of X1, X2 etc. to be estimated.

The implication of such a question is that the evaluator will be involved with structured approaches to data management, leading to an estimation of the extent of the causal link or links. This is consistent with a deductive approach to knowledge creation, and is often linked to the use of quantitative data collection and analysis methods. Such an approach is rooted in the canons of the so-called scientific method and has been used widely in some areas of the social sciences. In practice, such approaches have been adopted in evaluation studies, in particular within the Impact Form.

ANSWERING EVALUATION QUESTIONS

Evaluation questions are the basis for the evaluation design and the data management techniques that we employ. A distinguishing feature of evaluation practice is the need to have access to a repertoire of methods; to select and use data management techniques that are the most suitable for answering these questions. This is integral to the provision of plausible and accurate findings.

Figure 5.1 Data management in evaluation

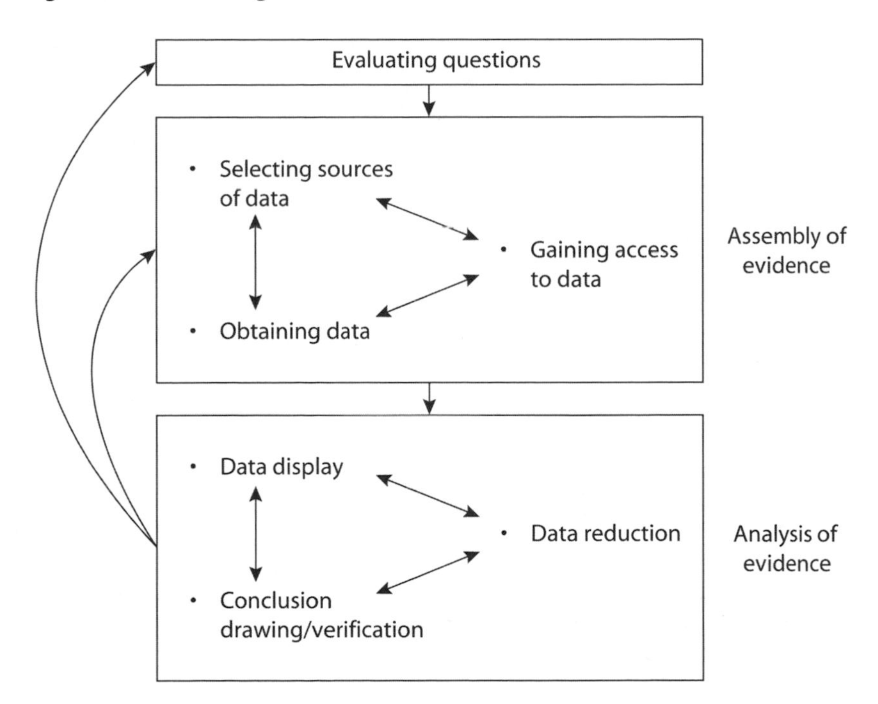

Figure 5.1 provides an overview of the link between asking for, and providing answers to, evaluation questions. Essential aspects of data management in evaluation include:

- the assembly of evidence—the collection of evidence relevant to each evaluation question; and
- analysis of evidence—making sense of these data through systematic data analysis techniques.

A large range of methods is available to evaluators. However, all these methods require the evaluator to be concerned with the elements of data collection and analysis that are outlined in Figure 5.1.

Assembly of evidence involves the following interlinked elements:

- *sources of data*—the actual location of the data, such as an existing file, documents, or individuals who possess the information required. This also involves the selection, where necessary, of data sources in instances where all relevant sources will not be consulted. Thus, sampling is a consideration in this element of data collection;
- *gaining access to data*—the means by which the data can be extracted. This involves making contact with data sources and involves aspects such as obtaining permission to consult with individuals, determining where and when data can be collected, and ensuring that ethical considerations are being observed; and
- *collecting data*—involving the development of instruments, and the use of these instruments to assemble evidence from the field. Instruments used in the collection of data include questionnaires, interviews and schemes for document review, as well as the methods used within them. For example, a given questionnaire might incorporate an attitude scale, a semantic differential scale, and an item that requires an extended written response.

Ways of assembling evidence can be summarized as follows:

- directly from individuals identified as sources of information:
  self-reports:
  - diaries or anecdotal records;
  - checklists or inventories;
  - rating scales and semantic differentials;
  - written responses;

  as personal products:
  - tests;
  - samples of work;
- compiled by an independent observer:
  written accounts;
  observation forms;

- observation schedules;
- rating scales;
- checklists and inventories;

oral responses, either singly or from a group;

- compiled by use of mechanical or electronic devices:
  audiotape;
  videotape;
  time-lapse and still photography;
  the Internet;
  - computer collation of responses;
- through use of unobtrusive techniques;
- from existing records:
  public documents;
  files;
  existing data bases or management information systems (MIS).

Analysis of evidence involves a consideration of the following interlinked elements:

- *data display*—the development of an organized assembly of information that leads to the drawing of conclusions about the key questions of the evaluation study;
- *data reduction*—the process of simplifying and transforming the raw information according to some logical set of procedures or rules;
- *conclusion drawing*—making meaning about the data in the terms of the question being examined.

It is possible that some studies will need more than one round of data collection and analysis to reach a conclusion. This explains the recursive arrow linking the conclusion drawing and verification element of data analysis back to the data collection stage in Figure 5.1.

As we have noted earlier, conclusion drawing is the end point of many evaluative inquiries. However, in others the evaluator may be concerned to use the conclusions to:

- *make judgments about the program*. This means placing values on the conclusions, such as making statements that the program is 'good' or 'bad', or that the results are 'positive', 'in the direction desired' or 'below expectations'.
- *develop recommendations*. These are suggested courses of action, advice to policy-makers, program managers or providers about what to do in light of the evidence and conclusions.

A detailed knowledge of specific data management techniques is beyond the scope of this book. Readers are encouraged to consult appropriate texts on individual techniques or to seek the assistance of an expert on technical matters of data analysis.

Numerous techniques for the analysis of data have been developed over time and have been made accessible to evaluators through sophisticated computer packages such as Statistical Packages for the Social Sciences (SPSS) and NVIVO. While these techniques vary in specifics, the above principles apply to them all. While it is true that canons or rules of data analysis for quantitative data are better specified and have stood the test of time, rules for the analysis of qualitative data have been developed which also fit within the principles described above (see for example, Miles and Huberman 1994).

It should also be noted that in all evaluations, a combination of common sense and an ability to be analytical can get the evaluator a long way towards conclusions on key evaluation issues or questions. If these attributes are used, it is possible to get by with some assistance from a methodological specialist at the 'right' time. We have continually been amazed at the quality of data management work done by graduate students if the above combination of factors has been present. This implies that the abilities of the evaluator are important in the collection and analysis of data.

An effective analyst needs specific mental powers *as well as* the relevant methodological tools (Maitland 1994, pp. 265–7). These mental powers include:

- the ability to *accumulate knowledge*—this involves the acquisition and synthesis of relevant information about the intervention under review;
- *observational abilities*—in terms of what to look for to recognize the meanings of the data and to be able to perceive and interpret available information;
- *reasoning powers*—the ability to build a line of argument or multiple lines of argument. This is consistent with the need to come to conclusions that can stand up to scrutiny;
- *intuitive powers*—the power of insight, the ability to make a conceptual leap in the face of lack of direct access to the phenomena of interest (Smith 1992).

As we have indicated earlier, the evaluation design is an integral part of evaluation planning and should be scrutinized before any fieldwork is undertaken. Designs should be subjected to the following pragmatic criteria:

- Will the evidence collected give a comprehensive picture of what is being evaluated?

- Does the data management strategy make effective use of existing data?
- Will the cost of data collection be justified, given the amount and kind of information it will provide?
- Will the information be reliable?
- Can the data collection be carried out without unduly disrupting the program and taking too much of the program providers' time?
- Are the data collection procedures legal and ethical?
- Can the data be collected and analyzed within the time constraints of the study?

This review may give the impression that data management proceeds in a linear and well-organized sequence of events. In practice, this is not the case. Data management involves a set of micro-level decisions, each one contingent on what has been decided before. Together these determine the direction of the analysis, and lead to the findings of the study. Consistent with the Emergent Realism paradigm is the desire of the conscientious evaluator to arrive as close to the truth as possible while retaining a sense of humility about the certainty of the conclusions made.

CONCLUSION

The fact that evaluation can no longer be regarded as a unitary concept is reflected in the different Forms of evaluation, each with identifiable purposes and issues that define them. Once the evaluator has determined which Forms are needed for a given evaluation, the next step is to develop appropriate evaluation questions.

We agree with Smith (1987) that fundamental to effective evaluation is good question development. This should be seen as the beginning of the vital data management aspect of evaluation practice. Clarifying evaluation questions assists clients and evaluators to see clearly what is needed, as well as helping to reject questions that are unanswerable and to put aside questions that are not important.

As we have emphasized, getting the key questions clear assists the evaluator in the selection of appropriate data management techniques. An effective evaluation is tightly focused, so the evaluator must be able to select and use efficient and effective methods. Chapters 9 to 13 are devoted to a discussion of evaluative inquiry for each of the evaluation Forms. These chapters contain case examples that provide a cross-section of the range of data management techniques available. Thus, while this chapter has provided an overview of methods, the material in later chapters should also contribute to your understandings of the use of these techniques.

REFERENCES

Datta, L. (1997). A pragmatic basis for mixed method designs. *New Directions for Program Evaluation*, 74 (Summer 1997), 33–46.

Greene, J. C. and Caracelli, V. J. (1997). Defining and describing the paradigm issue in mixed-method evaluation. *New Directions for Program Evaluation*, 74 (Summer 1997), 5–17.

Henry, G., Julnes, G. J. and Mark, M. M. (1998). Editor's Notes. *New Directions for Evaluation*, 78, 1–2.

Lambert, F. C., Owen, J. M., Coates, S. and McQueen, J. (1995). A guide to program evaluation. In *Professional Development for Program Evaluation*. Canberra, ACT: National Staff Development Committee for Vocational Education and Training.

Maitland, B. (1994). *The Marx Sisters*. Sydney: Allen & Unwin.

Meyer, H. (1997). *The Impact of the CSF in Schools*. Unpublished Doctor of Education thesis, The University of Melbourne.

Miles, M. B. and Huberman, A. M. (1994). *Qualitative Data Analysis*. Thousand Oaks, CA: Sage.

Owen, J. M., Meyer, H. and Livingston, J. (1996). *School Responses to the Curriculum and Standards Framework*. Carlton, Vic: Victorian Board of Studies.

Scriven, M. (1980). *The Logic of Evaluation*. Port Reyes, CA: Edge Press.

Smith, N. L. (1987). Towards the justification of claims in evaluation research. *Evaluation and Program Planning*, 10, 309–314.

Smith, N. L. (1992). Aspects of investigative inquiry in evaluation. *New Directions for Program Evaluation*, 56 (Winter), 3–13.

From Evaluation Findings to Utilization

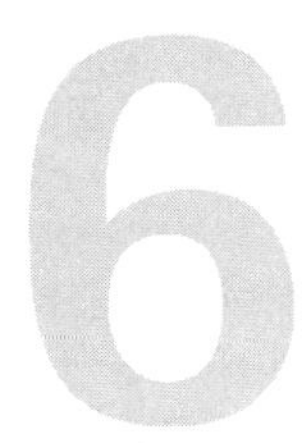

Evaluation use can be thought of as ways in which the findings of an evaluation influence the programs or policies that are the object of investigation, as well as affecting the organization within which an intervention is located. Evaluation use is of interest to public administrators and others who take the view that findings from systematic social inquiry should influence decision-making. Concern about evaluation use has been the subject of extensive debate among social scientists, reflecting a wider concern about the contributions of research to the economic and social advancement of countries that commit extensive resources to knowledge production in universities and allied institutions (Alkin & Taut 2003).

While use might, at first sight, seem to be a relatively simple construct, this has proved not to be the case in evaluation contexts. A key point of debate relates to *intentionality*. There are some who see use as the direct application of findings from a specific evaluation to the program under review in a one-to-one relationship. Michael Patton is among those who adopt this position. Then there are others who see use as more diffuse, so that decisions about a given program might draw on more than one evaluation finding. Carol Weiss is an example of those who hold this view. Extending this idea, the concept of *influence* has emerged, which takes into account indirect and multi-faceted applications of evaluation findings. Recently, scholars have attempted to draw together these various perspectives in order to present a unified theory of utilization to guide practice (see, for example, Johnson 1998; Kirkhart 2000).

EVALUATION TO UTILIZATION

From a review of the contributions of these and other theorists, we have developed a framework which summarizes key elements in the dissemination and utilization processes and presented in Figure 6.1. In this 'model', there are several major elements:

Figure 6.1 Conceptualizing evaluation utilization

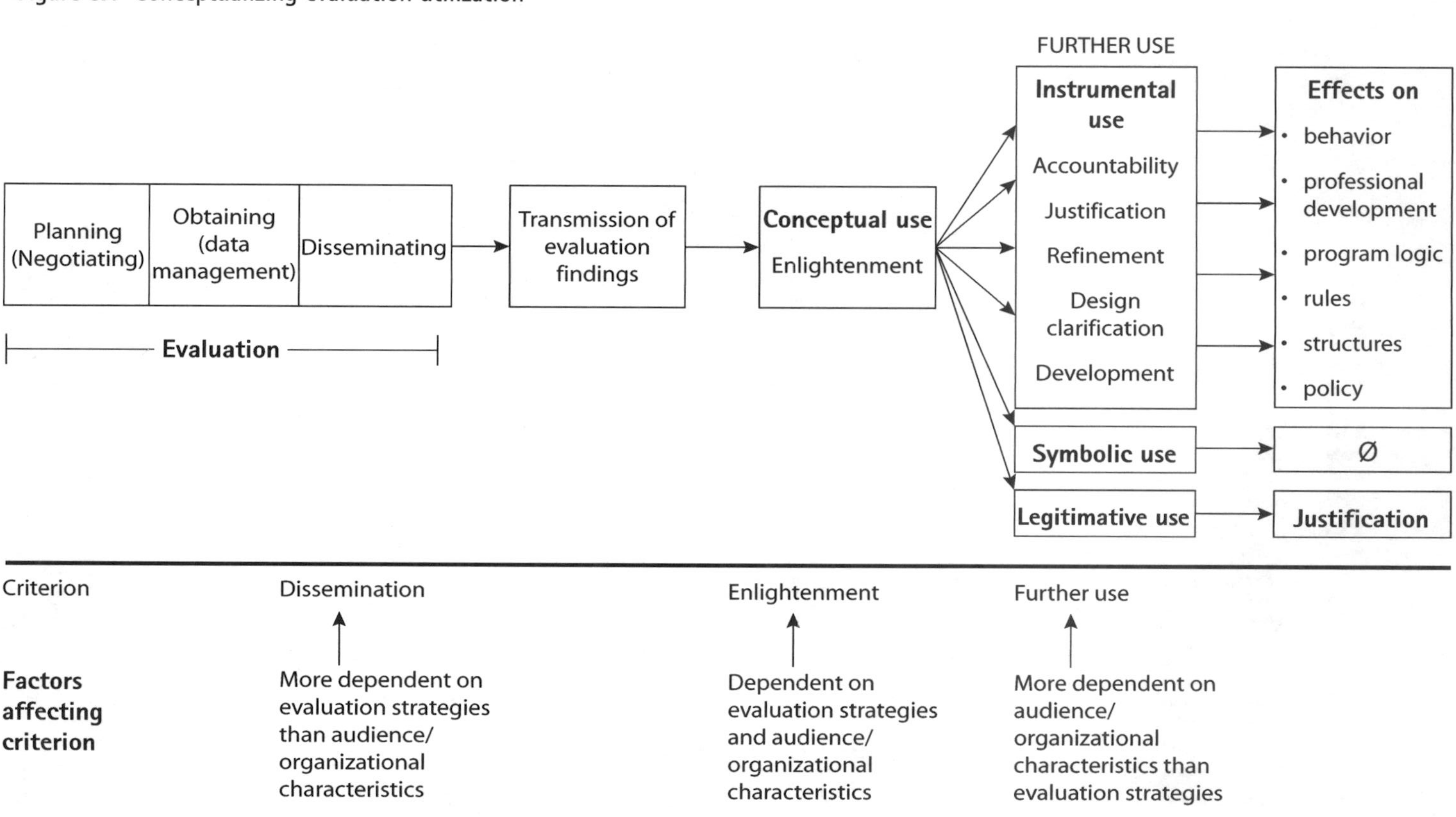

- *evaluation*, which consists of three key stages. As we have indicated previously, these are:
  - planning (and negotiation);
  - evaluation design—the assembly of evidence to produce findings; and
  - dissemination.

We have discussed the negotiating/planning and assembly of evidence and findings in previous chapters. Here, we focus on the following elements:

- *dissemination*—meaning the use of deliberative strategies and channels for informing identified audience(s) about aspects of the evaluation including its conduct and findings. While reporting of findings is an important and fundamental aspect it is not the only aspect of dissemination.

  The term 'dissemination' signifies that evaluators need to initiate strategies designed to encourage the spread of information resulting from the evaluation. Dissemination is used in preference to diffusion, the latter connoting a more general and less interventionist percolation of the findings to interested parties.
- *utilization*—an examination of Figure 6.1 reveals that there are, in conceptual terms, several stages of evaluation utilization. These are discussed below.

MEANINGS OF EVALUATION UTILIZATION

Utilization has a range of meanings, so we need to be clear about which meaning we adopt when discussing the impact of a given evaluation, or when we are concerned with encouraging the uptake of evaluation findings while in the negotiation and planning stage.

It is worthwhile spending a paragraph or two tracing the evolution of thinking about utilization. Early studies of the impact of an evaluation took a narrow definition that was based on direct observable effects, such as a policy change or the adoption of a new program initiative. Taking such a perspective, evidence of utilization would be in the direct and immediate impact of an evaluation on the program under review. This has been defined in the knowledge utilization literature as *instrumental use*, and refers to examples of an evaluation directly affecting decision-making, and in some cases actually influencing the program itself—for example, by a change in program implementation. Evidence of this type of utilization was sought in reported changes in decisions and actions that resulted from the evaluation, including the implementation of recommendations. The implication for studies of evaluation impact was that, if a given evaluation could not be seen to directly lead to instrumental use, that evaluation had not been utilized.

Based on an analysis of policy evaluations in the United States, Weiss (1999) encouraged an expansion of the notion of utilization to include *conceptual use*, or enlightenment. Conceptual use refers to cases where an evaluation is used to influence the thinking of the client about a program, but does not lead to decision-making related to the program. Weiss was influenced by her experience with policy-makers who valued findings from good evaluations which provided evidence about how their policies were being transformed into action in the field, and provided a basis for understanding what they were doing. Weiss also made the point that, over time, a series of evaluations could, cumulatively, affect decision-making about a major policy. Thus, while a series of individual evaluations had a conceptual impact, the sum of individual conceptual impacts could lead to an instrumental impact. This is the way policy changes often occur.

So, whereas evaluation impact was once judged solely in terms of effects on action, enlightenment was seen as an acceptable end point in the evaluation utilization chain. Enlightenment can help audiences to:

> understand the background and content of program operation, stimulate reverses of policy, focus attention on neglected issues, provide new understanding of the causes of social problems, clarify their own thinking, reorder priorities, make sense of what they have been doing, offer ideas for future directions, reduce uncertainties, create new uncertainties and provide rethinking of taken for granted assumptions, justify actions, support positions, persuade others, and provide a sense of how the world works (Weiss & Bucuavalas 1980, p. 136).

Those concerned about the impact of evaluations should not devalue enlightenment as a proper use of evaluations. This has been the case in the past, partly because conceptual use had not been accepted as utilization. Also, enlightenment impact has been difficult to measure and studies of conceptual use have been open to charges that they are 'less objective' than measures which are linked to action.

It should also be noted that the findings of any one evaluation can also add to the knowledge base about a given research issue—that is, evaluation findings can be seen as contributing to our understanding of important educational and social phenomena. There are some evaluators who see a contribution to what could be called 'funded knowledge' as their primary role. However, others would argue that when the primary purpose of a given investigation is to add to the scientific knowledge base, rather than respond to the agenda of stakeholders, such investigations are more aptly described as 'applied research'.

In the context of policy research, enlightenment has been dissected into three phases as follows:

- *Reception.* Utilization takes place when policy-makers or advisers receive policy-relevant information. When the communication comes to rest in the 'in-basket' so that the data reach the policy-maker rather than remain on an analyst's desk or in the in-files of a distant consultant firm, reception has occurred.
- *Cognition.* The policy-maker must read, digest and understand the study for cognition to occur.
- *Reference.* If frame of reference is the criterion, then utilization somehow must change the way the policy-maker sees the world. If information changes his or her preferences or understandings of the probabilities of magnitudes of impacts she or he fears or desires, utilization is a reality. Altering frames of reference is important because, in the long run, the policy-maker's new vision will emerge in different policy priorities (Knott & Wildavsky 1980, p. 303).

This suggests that evaluators can play an educative role—that is, audiences learn about their program via an evaluative inquiry, both at the individual and organizational level. The evaluator facilitates increased understanding of the design or implementation of a program or how an organization is working. This might involve an evaluator working inside an organization that is committed to learning about the way it operates. In a study of trends in evaluation use among members of the American Evaluation Association, it was shown that there has been a large increase in evaluations which had such an emphasis (Preskill & Caracelli 1996).

These views about utilization resulted from vigorous debate about the influence of evaluations, and of what can be expected of evaluators in terms of the impact of their work. The kind of utilization that could be expected depends on a range of factors, not least of which is the nature of the intervention and the Form of evaluation selected. If an evaluator is working closely with provider staff 'on the ground' in the Interactive Form, one might normally expect that a well-conducted evaluation would directly influence the program instrumentally. This is the position Patton takes in his developmental evaluation approach (Patton 1997). Alternatively, at the 'Big P' or policy level, research suggests that most evaluations can only expect to enlighten audiences. However, we have been involved in managing large-scale evaluation studies where particular attention was given to instrumental use. For example, in early 2005 a government announced changes to national policy on homelessness that resulted directly from a report that was tabled less than six months before. This was an evaluation where extensive attempts were made to keep policy-makers informed of the findings of the evaluation and their implications for practice (Wyatt et al. 2004).

We have taken these meanings of utilization into account and added a couple of additional ones to prepare a 'model' of utilization in which the first stage in utilization is that the audience becomes enlightened (Figure 6.1).

Enlightenment means:

- knowledge of the plan and conduct of the evaluation; and
- comprehension of the findings.

Enlightenment can be the end point of the utilization chain. A decision as to whether the enlightenment or educative aspect is to be the end point should be made in the planning/negotiation phase of a given study.

In some evaluations, enlightenment is the first stage leading to 'further use'. Further use occurs when findings are applied to the program under review in some way. Evaluations themselves cannot make such applications, so it is necessary for someone to link the information from an evaluation to the existing condition of the program under review. Nevertheless, to engage in rational action, it is necessary for the audience to become enlightened about what has been found during the evaluation. We therefore contend that in *all* evaluations, whether the end point is to be enlightenment or some kind of further use, it is incumbent on the evaluator to adopt communication strategies that will inform the audience to the utmost about the findings of the evaluation. This leads back to the need for evaluators to be good communicators and to plan suitable dissemination strategies to ensure that audiences have a high conceptual grasp of the salient outcomes of a given evaluation study.

Three broad possibilities of further use are suggested in Figure 6.1. One possibility is that findings from a given evaluation may be used for legitimative purposes—that is, to justify decisions already made about the program. Thus, the evaluation follows decision-making, and provides a way of retrospectively justifying decisions made on other grounds, and responds to a concern of the policy-maker for support. Muscatello (1988) defends the legitimative use of evaluation as part of the work of an evaluation unit in an organization. The circumstance is that:

> the decision has already been made and the evaluation unit is asked to develop data or undertake work which can verify or legitimize the decision (which usually would not be common organizational knowledge until the evaluation effort was complete). When the decision becomes public, an implementation plan is drawn up. This

can be a particularly sensitive area for an evaluation manager, who may be required to (a) bring to the attention of the decision maker any data which conflict with the proposed decision, and (b) resolve the conflicts. If resolution is not possible, the final report may have to be structured in such a way that the decision is palatable to the rest of the organization.

Purists in the evaluation field may take exception to this, considering a verification evaluation not to be an evaluation at all. Pragmatists, however, may be justified in observing that such an effort is nevertheless a valid function of an evaluation unit (p. 32).

A second possibility is symbolic use. This is consistent with an evaluation being commissioned by an individual or a group that has no interest in applying the results. The commissioner may be going through the motions to satisfy the need for an evaluation as part of a contract with the program-funding agency. Or the commissioner has ulterior motives—for example, using involvement in an evaluation process to curry favor with a superior, for career advancement, or to include involvement in the evaluation on a *vita*. In symbolic use, no modifications to the existing program follow from the dissemination of evaluation findings.

While some would cavil at these possibilities being counted as utilization at all, Pelz (1978) believes that these two types once represented the dominant usage in complex organizations: 'in the domain of policy making, one suspects that symbolic or legitimative use may be more prevalent than conceptual use with instrumental use appearing rarely' (p. 350).

A third possible further use is that evaluation findings provide a basis for action. This is instrumental use, introduced earlier in this chapter. In practice, instrumental use can take on a range of meanings that will vary from evaluation to evaluation. Instrumental use may mean making decisions about:

- developing a program;
- clarifying an existing program design;
- refining a program in action;
- justifying the approaches used; or
- accounting for the resources spent on developing and implementing the intervention.

These are consistent with the orientation of different Forms of evaluative inquiry.

Associated with the instrumental type of further use are alternative actions. As indicated in Figure 6.1, actions could include changes in one or more of the following:

- program logic;
- program delivery—that is, behavioral changes in people;
- rules of the organization which is responsible for the program;
- structures of this organization;
- the philosophy or mission of the organization.

In the lower half of Figure 6.1, key criterion variables in the utilization chain are linked to the influences of key players in the evaluation paradigm. Experience and a brief review of the literature suggest that, along the chain, there is a shift in responsibility for the success of each stage. This is summarized in the following generalizations:

- *Dissemination* is highly dependent on evaluator efforts to be responsive to audience needs during the conduct of the evaluation. Dissemination is less dependent on 'openness to change' characteristics of the audience/organization for whom the evaluation is intended.
- *Enlightenment* is highly dependent on evaluator efforts to be responsive to audience needs during the conduct of the evaluation, and on the communication strategies used in the study. 'Openness to change' characteristics of the audience/organization will also affect the extent of enlightenment.
- *Further use*, particularly instrumental use, is highly dependent on 'openness to change' characteristics of the audience/organization for whom the evaluation findings are intended. It is less dependent on evaluator efforts to be responsive to audience needs in planning and during the conduct of the evaluation.

PROCESS USE

While this section has emphasized that the findings of an evaluation are fundamental to utilization, Smith (1988) suggests that the *act* of evaluation can in itself stimulate thinking and change in an organization responsible for a program. This can occur when the evaluator is an insider, or where the evaluator works closely and cooperatively in conjunction with organizational groups who actually participate in the evaluation process (Patton 2003, p. 230). In this case the dissemination of information about the evaluation happens continuously during the evaluation and leads to significant learning. Benefits accrue to program providers and other stakeholders by having an opportunity to interact with those who evaluate their program. This is over and above the use of evaluation findings by these providers in the ways described above. An implication here is that, due to the fact that an evaluation is being conducted, there will be changes in individuals or organizations.

This has been defined as process use, which:

> refers to the cognitive and behavioral changes resulting from users' engagement in the evaluation process. Process use occurs when those involved in the evaluation learn from the evaluation process—as, for example, when those involved in the evaluation later say, 'The impact on our program came not so much from the findings as from going through the thinking process that the evaluation required' (Preskill & Caracelli 1996, p. 13).

A desired outcome of process use is for providers to absorb the skills and ways of thinking that evaluators use routinely. This encourages providers to think in different ways about what they do, with a more critical edge. It is assumed that this will lead to more effective program delivery and organizational health. In the longer term, such experiences help engender an evaluation culture within an organization and encourage providers to engage in their own evaluation work. In this sense, process use can lead to subsequent investigations in which instrumental use and program improvement become routine in organizations.

Example 6.1 Evaluation as a stimulus for review

An external evaluator assisted a federal agency to develop an evaluation resource that was used by each of its seventeen regional offices to undertake a self-review of recent projects. While the findings were of importance for each region, it was found that the processes of developing the resource for the evaluation acted as a strategy for sensitizing regional committees to a range of current educational issues. Taking part in the resource development and subsequent evaluations was the means by which regional committees came to grips with recent policy developments. It also forced them to become more in touch with their constituents, in this case families and community groups within each region.

FACTORS AFFECTING UTILIZATION

To this point, we have provided a conceptual map of utilization. We now turn to considering factors *affecting* utilization (see Figure 6.2). This section is based on the utilization literature, for example, a major empirical review (Cousins & Leithwood 1986), and a more recent analysis of the impact of evaluation on policy decision-making (Weiss 1999).

Figure 6.2 Simple utilization paradigm

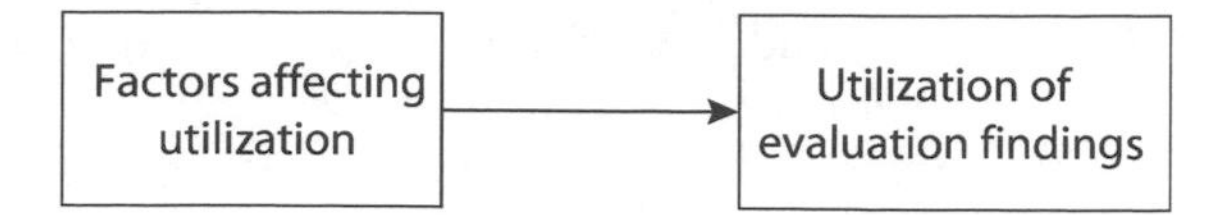

By and large, these studies classify factors affecting utilization into two clusters; relating to the:

- characteristics of the evaluation—that is, the way that the evaluation is conducted; and
- characteristics of the setting in which the findings are to be utilized—that is, factors nested in the organization which has commissioned the evaluation.

Characteristics of the evaluation

Cousins and Leithwood (1986) discuss six factors which were shown to affect utilization. With reference to Figure 6.2, four factors relate mainly to the conduct of the evaluative inquiry. These are:

- relevance;
- credibility;
- quality; and
- findings.

The other two relate mainly to dissemination. These are:

- communication; and
- timeliness of reporting.

Relevance of evaluation information can be thought of as the degree to which the evaluation was focused on issues relevant to the audience. This implies the identification of primary users and their major concerns during the negotiation phase of the evaluation. There is considerable evidence, particularly at the policy level, that evaluation results will be used to the extent that they are relevant to the issues and interests of the management decision-maker. At this level, Lipton (1992) exhorts one to:

> stay focused on the critical policy relevant questions. Evaluation results have to compete in a political decision-making arena with other weighty desiderata. Focusing on critical issues improves the chances that evaluation results will have an impact. The more undifferentiated

'nice-to-know' material added to the body, the less likely the evaluation report will be utilized and have an impact (p. 182).

Credibility refers to the characteristics of the evaluator and the degree to which the evaluator is credible and believable. While the evidence is variable, there is a trend for utilization to be linked to an evaluator being an impartial and creditable practitioner. Key attributes include:

- competence and record of successful evaluation work;
- objectivity, credibility and bias;
- specialization of skills;
- being able to undertake evaluation for minimum cost;
- being flexible and able to use methods which are responsive to the needs of individual evaluations.

In summary, there must be user trust in the evaluator. Conley-Tyler (2005) suggests that the greatest differences between internal and external evaluators lie in the areas of evaluator objectivity and accountability. Whereas external evaluators are seen to bring these aspects with them, internal evaluators only gain respect over time through a history of productive evaluations that impress the employer.

Quality refers to the conduct of the data management phase—such as the choice of methods and the rigor by which the data are collected and analyzed. One could think of this as being the research component of evaluative inquiry. Research quality was reported as being important to utilization across nearly half of the studies examined by Cousins and Leithwood.

Findings include the nature of results, the implications for decision-making, and their relationship to the concerns of the audiences. Evaluations must be able to produce relevant and timely information for a given situation. Users must believe what evaluators have to say—that is, the findings must make sense. Weiss and Bucuavalas (1980) showed that decision-makers faced with findings on an issue applied two criteria, a truth test and a utility test, when assessing the potential usefulness of the research to their circumstances. Note that this is one of the few studies where conceptual use is the criterion variable.

Dimensions of truth were:

- research quality—the scientific merit of the investigation; and
- conformity to user expectations—the consistency between the findings and what the reader knows about the subject.

Dimensions of utility were:

- action orientation—the practicability of the findings contained in the research; and
- challenge to the status quo—the extent to which the findings provide information in conflict with the current policies and operations of the organization or system.

All four variables explained variations in the usefulness of the findings, with research quality having the greatest effect. The analysis also found that a negative interaction existed between the two truth dimensions—that is, the less the findings conformed to the previous ideas of the decision-maker, the more it was necessary for the findings to have resulted from sound research (and vice versa). There was also a negative correlation between the utility scales—that is, if a study challenged the status quo it was not so important for it to be action orientated.

Moving on to the final two factors affecting utilization, and relating to dissemination:

Communication refers to the quality and quantity of communication during the evaluation study, the clarification of information when necessary, and the advocacy of the results. Research has shown a clear and strong relationship between the quality of communication between decision-makers and evaluators and the use of evaluation findings, particularly during the evaluation process. We discuss communication more inclusively in the section on dissemination later in the chapter.

Timeliness refers to the provision of findings and other products from an evaluation in time to meet the decision needs of the audience. Reviews suggest that timeliness is positively related to utilization; it is difficult to envisage how it could be negatively related, as studies that do not deliver on time are less likely to be considered. Poor timing can limit or preclude use of evaluation findings; evaluation findings presented at opportune times are more likely to influence decision-makers.

Characteristics of the setting which affect utilization

As we have indicated, the organizational setting in which the audience for the evaluation is situated has a major impact on the extent to which the evaluation findings are used in conceptual or instrumental ways. Cousins and Leithwood (1986) and Hudson-Mabbs (1993) identified six organizational factors that affect utilization. These are:

- commitment;
- information needs/competing information;
- personal characteristics;

- decision-making;
- political climate; and
- financial climate.

Commitment relates to features such as audience participation and attitudes towards the role of evaluation in program and policy change. Many studies have shown a link between commitment and knowledge use. There is an assumption that, through involvement in negotiation and planning, audience commitment can be developed or enhanced. For example, Greene (1988) found that audience participation in evaluation increased the likelihood that the findings of the evaluation would be used.

Commitment needs to be built through the negotiation of an appropriate plan that is acceptable to clients and evaluation commissioners (Owen et al. 1994). Generally, this means a plan that they have sanctioned. Giving the primary audience a say in the plan increases the chances of the evaluators asking salient questions. If the scope of an evaluation is too narrow, utilization could be minimal because the findings do not address substantive issues. Negotiation also helps set realistic time limits and encourages the use of reporting methods which can be comprehended by the audiences.

Negotiation contributes more towards utilization than merely agreeing on an evaluation plan. Interaction between evaluator and client within the negotiation process can build up personal and professional rapport between them. Personal rapport means that evaluator and client enjoy each other's company and are able to extend that compatibility to their discussion of evaluation matters. Professional rapport is more task-oriented and is manifested in a shared interest in the nature of the program and the means used to evaluate it. These forms of rapport are often found together and, when they are, the likelihood of utilization of evaluation information is enhanced. Put simply, the involvement of potential users in the planning stage is designed to build the commitment of the users.

In some evaluations, the line between program and evaluation components can be blurred. There may be instances when the term 'evaluation' is never mentioned. For example, in some Approaches in the Interactive Form—such as action research—the integration of evaluation with program delivery makes sense for several reasons. The first is that it increases the chance of obtaining good data if the participants perceive that the evaluative component can also make a contribution to their learning (Preskill & Torres 2000). For example, in evaluating a training program the evaluators may ask participants to reflect on the knowledge base they bring to the training. They may also be asked to explain why they came to the training and what they expected to learn. These data can serve as a 'pre-test'—as a baseline for collecting post-course data. Second, program/evaluation interaction can reduce the cost of evaluation if it can be incorporated into proceedings. For example, it may be possible for the data collection to be administered by program staff. Third, this approach is likely to increase the chances of the findings being useful to the program staff and administration.

Example 6.2 Evaluation of supervision training

In an evaluation of a supervision training program conducted by a state Community Services Department, we worked closely with program deliverers to develop a plan in which the evaluation data collection was part of the program. In the first session, participants were asked to complete a short form which listed their present levels of knowledge on key supervision issues, and their reasons for attending the program. This was immediately used by deliverers and participants as a means of refining the goals and procedures of the program. This information was also used as a basis for collecting information on the immediate impact of the program and on changes to participant performance in the workplace (Owen & McLeod 1991).

In the context of increasing the use of evaluations conducted by internal evaluators, Muscatello (1988) believes that the determination of evaluation priorities is a first step to increasing commitment to the use of findings. He developed a difficulty rating procedure and grid for determining which of competing evaluation proposals should proceed to implementation. In the same context of internal evaluation, Mowbray (1988) suggests that there are six steps for maximizing utilization findings. These are:

- marketing evaluation as a worthwhile service;
- developing and focusing policy questions;
- planning and designing the evaluation;
- conducting the evaluation;
- translating the findings; and
- making people pay attention to the evaluation results.

It is worth noting that the many evaluators would see the first and last steps as being outside the boundaries of their responsibility. This may be because most of the debate about utilization assumes that the evaluator is externally based. Mowbray says that, when an evaluator is internal to the organization, there is a need to remind others continually of the benefits of evaluation findings in decision-making. Mowbray and others suggest that internal evaluators are well placed to increase impact, at least to the enlightenment stage of use.

Example 6.3 Making a difference in decision-making

In an evaluation of competing programs or streams within a postgraduate course in teacher education, an internally-based evaluation group played a strong role in decisions about the future of the competing programs. This was possible because the evaluation team was known to the stakeholders, the steering committee sponsoring the evaluation, and had established a practice of interacting with them throughout the study. There was attention to dissemination throughout the study as well as the transmission of the findings. In terms of further use, the evaluators were influential in overturning a decision in-principle to axe one program which was difficult to administer and more costly to implement. The evaluation findings showed clearly that this program was educationally superior. Evidence that supported this claim was personally presented at steering committee meetings. The evaluators were on site and 'on tap' to interact with key decision-makers during a crucial period of negotiation about the future of the programs (Owen 1984).

There may also be instances where an internal evaluator takes up the responsibility for instrumental use of the evaluation, by having at least a partial say in the decision-making which follows an evaluation. For example, after an evaluation of a major program in a large secondary school, one of the evaluation team agreed to attend meetings of the school's program-planning committee. He provided advice to the committee on a regular basis on matters related to the evaluation and its implications for changing the school curriculum (Owen et al. 1994).

Information needs relates to the perceived need for relevant knowledge and the types of information that audiences turn to for decision-making and problem-solving. It has been found that the more an organization adopts a 'climate of rationality' (Weiss 1999) and looks outwards for new knowledge, the more likely it will turn to evaluation and use evaluation findings. Associated with this is *competing information*, which refers to alternative sources of information. Several writers have found that the existence of additional information about a program—for example, the experiences of opinion leaders—is an important factor influencing the use of findings from a given evaluation. This is particularly so in the case of policy evaluation.

Evaluation findings are generally used in conjunction with other credible sources, such as information provided by advisers—sources that have proven more useful than those from evaluations (Alkin & Dalliak 1985).

Personal characteristics refer to the attitudes of individuals towards evaluation and their influence and experience within organizations. Patton (1997) has documented in detail the role of a significant individual in influencing the application of findings to program change and improvement. Characteristics of such an individual include leadership, interest, enthusiasm, determination, aggressiveness and access to power. In government, this has been recognized for some time; in a review of evaluation use in government it was noted that:

> over and over again, the most important factor in assuring the use of evaluation findings was not the quality of the evaluation but the existence of a decision maker who wants and needs an evaluation and has committed himself to implementing its findings (Chelimsky 1977).

The implications for the planning stage is that evaluators need to identify a significant individual or group who has the inclination and the power to use the findings—should they be judged adequate—in program decision-making. Alkin and colleagues (1979) suggest the following categories:

- people who can use the information;
- people for whom the information makes a difference;
- people who have questions they want answered;
- people who care and are willing to share responsibility for the evaluation and its utilization.

In some cases there is an individual person or small group of people within an organization, which is the key to further use. While this entity is sometimes the commissioner of the evaluation, in other instances this will be not be the case. For example, in a nationally funded evaluation of university/college-based pre-service teacher education programs, the steering committee decided that faculty of the appropriate departments of the colleges were to be the primary audience for the study. This was in recognition that these staff would have the major responsibility for implementing recommendations from the evaluation (Owen et al. 1985).

Decision-making refers to the context in which decisions about the program are made, and the type of decision to be made. Cousins and Leithwood (1986) found this was a constant factor affecting utilization across studies. As we have seen, a range of decisions can be linked to the instrumental use of evaluation findings. Clearly there is a difference between what might be called *retrospective* decisions for justification or accountability reasons, and *prospective* decisions—for example, to develop or modify a program. The type of decision that is likely to be made should be identified in the planning stage; research suggests that such a strategy will increase the chance of utilization.

Political climate includes the existing political orientation of the organization. There is a greater likelihood that evaluation findings will be used if they are consistent with the existing political realities which impinge on the organization. Empirical studies reviewed by Cousins and Leithwood (1986) found that evaluation utilization was politically influenced at both the organizational and extra-organizational levels.

Financial climate relates to the current level of support for the program under review and for changes suggested by the evaluation. There is some evidence that where findings suggest changes that involve only moderate costs, as distinct from high costs, findings are more likely to be adopted. The presence of this factor reminds us that it is incumbent on evaluators to give considerations to the financial implications of their findings wherever possible.

In considering this section, we must emphasize that these findings have been drawn from diverse studies, most of which have used instrumental use as their criterion. That is, very few studies have attempted to measure conceptual use. We also draw attention to the interactive nature of the variables that lead to use, and the fact that few, if any, studies have been able to look at multiple causes of use. Finally, we believe that use is contextual: what influences use in one setting will not be important in another. The major use of this review should be to alert those who are planning evaluations to the possible factors that will affect use in their own setting. These should be considered carefully in the planning and negotiation phase of the evaluation and reviewed throughout the study.

Finally, we include some generalizations from our own experience in evaluation practice which suggest the following:

- The more the evaluator consults with audiences during the planning phase, the more the findings will be used.
- The more the evaluator pursues questions of importance to the audiences, the more the findings will be used.
- The more interactive the communication, the more the findings will be used.
- The less complex the mix of audiences, the more the findings will be used.
- The more proximate the evaluator is to the audiences throughout the evaluation, the more likely the findings will be used.

- The more assistance the evaluator provides with implementation of the findings, the more the findings will be used.
- Any evaluator who thinks his or her study will have an exclusive impact on change in the program or organization under review is suffering from delusion.

DISSEMINATION AND REPORTING

Dissemination involves strategies and channels designed to inform audiences about relevant aspects of an evaluation. In a well-executed evaluation, the client is kept informed about all aspects of the study. For this to occur, channels of communication must be kept open throughout. Dissemination relies on dialogue between stakeholders and their audiences. For example, towards the end of a study, there may be merit in promoting opportunities for an open-ended two-way communication through which findings of the evaluation and associated implications for action are explored, rather than being provided as recommendations by the evaluators.

Findings

As indicated in Chapter 1, findings include the following:

- *evidence*—the data and other information which has been collected during the evaluation;
- *conclusions*—the synthesis of data and information. These are the meanings made by those involved in the evaluation through the synthesis of data. This involves evaluators in the processes of data display, data reduction and verification;
- *judgments*—in which values are placed on the conclusions. Criteria are applied to the conclusions stating that the program is 'good' or 'bad', or that the results are 'positive', 'in the direction desired' or 'below expectations'; and
- *recommendations*—suggested courses of action, advice to policy-makers, program managers or providers about what to do in the light of the evidence and conclusions.

All evaluation involves the collection and analysis of evidence and the reaching of conclusions. However, there will be variations from study to study in the degree to which findings incorporate the making of judgments or recommendations. In some Forms—for example, those within the Proactive evaluation Form—there will be little concern with making judgments in a traditional sense. In this case, the evaluator's role could stop at the conclusion-drawing stage.

Some studies will include recommendations, others will not. Whether or not recommendations are included should be negotiated during the planning stage of the evaluation. It should be noted that recommendations relate to what needs to be done in the future, while most other findings relate to what is or what has been.

> Philosophically, evaluators should view the evaluation findings (conclusions) as an accurate description of the conditions they have encountered, and not subject to change. Recommendations, on the other hand, are crafted by the evaluators and program staff, and are subject to judgment and interpretation of the data. Conceptually, recommendations are judgments by evaluators based on the findings of the report about changes in program activities that are likely to bring about some desired future condition. Shedding the retrospective role of evaluation, the writer of the recommendations looks forward, proposing activities that are expected to improve program effectiveness (Sonnichsen 1994, p. 542).

Recent research into the nature of recommendations suggests that evaluators should pay more attention to their creation and presentation to audiences. There is a mistaken belief that 'offering recommendations is a straightforward and simple process that flows naturally from the conclusions of an evaluation' (Hendricks 1994, p. 558).

Following an analysis of the use of recommendations in a State audit office, Sharma (2004) developed guidelines that are designed to address the issues that were raised by Hendricks, as follows:

- clients or users should be involved in developing recommendations as much as possible. This implies that clients must be aware of what has been found during the study. This strategy is likely to result in recommendations that are: understandable, directed to appropriate persons or groups, appropriate to the context, and are feasible and practical;
- not all recommendations are created equally. Evaluators should identify differences in the recommendations they offer, in that some require greater effort and encouragement to adopt than others. In other words, evaluators need to understand how the nature of their recommendations will influence the likelihood of their adoption and utilization. Some recommendations are more directly 'usable' than others;
- evaluators need to consider how recommendations are to be conveyed, and be active in encouraging clients to adopt them (Sharma 2004, pp. 143–146).

More explicitly, and based on a contribution by Hendricks and Papagiannis (1990), the list below provides guidance for making effective recommendations.

- Use the planning/negotiation stage to determine whether recommendations are part of the findings.
- If recommendations are to be made, decide who is to make them—evaluators or clients or evaluators/clients working together.
- Consider all issues to be 'fair game' for recommendations.
- Don't wait until the end of the evaluation to begin thinking about recommendations.
- Link recommendations to the evidence where possible.
- Work closely with clients throughout the evaluation.
- Consider the contexts in which the recommendations will be implemented.
- Offer only realistic recommendations.
- Decide how specific the recommendations are to be.
- Think twice about recommending fundamental changes.
- Outline the future implications of your recommendations.
- Make the recommendations easy to understand.
- If possible, stay involved after the recommendations have been accepted.
- If a recommendation is not accepted, look for other opportunities to recommend it again.

We have found that interspersing recommendations, or in some cases 'issues for consideration', within the text of an evaluation report provides the link some readers need to establish the credibility of the findings. The following example is a paragraph from an evaluation report of the school-level use of educational resources commissioned by a national research organization. It was written when reviewing the evidence on the internal school distribution of newsletters and other materials which come into schools from this organization.

Example 6.4 'Issues for consideration' within an evaluation report

Across the more active schools, there seems to be two sequential steps. The first involves the Principal distributing the newsletter to other senior staff—for example, the curriculum coordinator, deputy principal, etc. Another ploy is for the Principal to send it to a specific staff member who has an interest in the material covered by the newsletter. Another strategy is to send it to the librarian, to a teacher resource or professional development section. A small proportion of schools routinely discuss newsletter issues at staff meetings. The second step involves deposition of the newsletter in a consolidated location, presumably for future reference. This could be the teacher reference section in the library, a rack or similar in the staff room. In other schools there is a filing system kept by a senior member of staff.

Issue for consideration
Some intensive studies of exemplary school internal information dissemination which focused on other resources besides the newsletter, including materials for the classroom, would be useful for the research organization to establish more effective ways of presenting information for dissemination (Owen et al. 1996).

All 'issues for consideration' were also included in an executive summary at the beginning of the report.

Styles of reporting

While it was once the norm for evaluators to rely on a major end-of-study written report as the major style of reporting, concerns about the lack of impact of this strategy has led to an examination of alternative forms of communication.

In reporting findings, issues which need to be decided include:

- strategies for reporting;
- types of reports; and
- effective ways of presenting material within these reports.

Strategies

As discussed earlier in this chapter, timely dissemination is critical, as decision-makers must have the information when it is required. There is little point in executing an elegant evaluation design if the findings are too late to influence decisions about the program.

It is not always possible to anticipate the timing of the information needs of audiences. In some cases evaluators must release information in response to audience requests before the final analyses are complete. There is then a need to compromise between completeness and utility. Our view is that requests for information should be responded to with the clear caveat that the information is the 'best available' at the time the request was made. Good evaluators build in to the evaluation design strategies which will allow dissemination in installments rather than as a single end-of-evaluation tome. This implies that an evaluation can be divided into defined stages, each with its own products and findings.

There are advantages, in terms of audience comprehension, in reporting information in a series of smaller chunks rather than in a monolithic report at the conclusion of the project. An audience is more likely to read smaller reports, and to absorb the essential messages, than they would if they were presented within a large report. In the case of reports to management, there is evidence that, due to work pressures, bureaucrats find it difficult to absorb large amounts of complex information. In addition, serial reporting allows for the release of specific information which may be required at different times. There is also an advantage in that smaller reports spread the workload of evaluator document preparation. A disadvantage, on the other hand, is that findings of the study may appear fragmented if reported over time, and it is sometimes necessary to adopt some form of overview document to minimize this. It is also possible that many—if not most—of the salient findings will not be known until near the end of the evaluation.

Types of reports

When planning dissemination strategies, evaluators should take into account the following dimensions. Options here include:

- written versus oral;
- progress versus final;
- substantive (main report) versus secondary (such as technical details of data management);
- summary versus main report;
- formal versus informal;
- descriptive versus recommendatory.

Formats

Possible formats of written reports include acceptable professional writing and less formal styles, perhaps without referencing and composed in a more vernacular style. There is some evidence that interactive reporting and the use of strategies other than formal reports increases the chances of audience utilization of evaluation findings. Quotations designed to highlight key findings can also be embedded within the body of the report. There may also be merit in using briefer reports. Examples suggested by Macy (1981) include:

- evaluation briefs at the end of main reports;
- an executive summary;
- 'googles'—these are one-liners designed to make members of the audience appear intelligent and well read.

In addition to written reports, other forms of presentation such as oral reports, displays and photography/videos may be used. Displays in the form of graphs and charts can summarize and present large amounts of information in an attractive way.

The detail of reporting will vary from evaluation to evaluation and should be negotiated in the planning stage of a study. Generally, a combination of reporting methods is necessary to take into account the needs of different audiences.

EFFECTS ON ACTION

The ultimate in the evaluation utilization chain presented in Figure 6.1 is the effects of evaluation findings on action. This means improvements in programs and policies. At a societal level, a goal of evaluation has been seen as the achievement of social betterment (Henry & Mark 2003). At the organizational level Downs (1967) suggested that action which results from evaluation can be grouped into four clusters:

- *behavior*—changes in the conduct of an organization's members bringing them closer to the way they would behave if they were totally in agreement with the organization's goals;
- *rules*—changes in the organization's formal procedures covering how employees should act in producing the organization's products or services;
- *structures*—changes involving the hierarchy containing the distributions of power, information and prestige among the members of the organization;
- *purpose* or *raison d'être*—changes in the fundamental values underlying the goals and actions of an organization.

Using Downs' categories, (Johnston 1988) undertook an analysis of recommendations made in evaluations conducted by the US General Accounting Office (GAO). He found that the majority of recommendations were related to changes in behavior and that these were more likely to have been implemented than those in the other three categories. The implication is that organizational processes are more likely to be addressed within evaluation than more substantive aspects of the functioning of organizations, a finding that has more recently been endorsed by Sharma (2004).

The transition from enlightenment to action and change is an area where evaluators have traditionally not involved themselves. However, there is patently a need for assistance with change *per se*, and if change to programs and organizations based on evaluations is to take place, then the evaluator is a candidate to assist with the implementation of the change effort. This has been an increasing feature of the practice of evaluators who are being asked to facilitate change in agencies which have adopted a learning organization focus.

Example 6.5 Implementing change arising from evaluation findings

In a review of the middle school program of a large inner-city high school, the evaluation recommended that the program should be completely overhauled and linked more closely to the curriculum offered before and afterwards, up and down the school. Consequent to the dissemination of findings to the school, one of the evaluators worked continuously to implement these findings, a process that took almost two years before all the recommendations were implemented.

Based on this study we proposed four major principles for evaluation practice which adopted an 'effects on action focus'. These included:

- negotiation of a plan which is acceptable to stakeholders;
- heightening awareness about the evaluation by making data collection procedures visible to stakeholders;
- using interactive and timely synergistic techniques of reporting; and
- providing guidelines and ongoing personal-level support for the implementation of findings (Owen et al. 1994).

The inclusion of the fourth of these principles implies that evaluators should possess knowledge about organizational change and implementation theory, and skills in working with practitioners to implement changes that are suggested by the evaluation. Evaluators are in a unique position to assist stakeholders to maximize the instrumental use of findings. If the evaluator has sound human relations skills, he or she is uniquely placed to encourage an informed and balanced use of the findings. Such use by the stakeholders, acting alone, cannot always be guaranteed—evaluation findings can often be misinterpreted by those to whom they are directed. Our view is that evaluation findings have a much greater chance of impacting on action if the evaluator takes on the role of change consultant (Owen & Lambert 1995). This has particular implications for the creation of positions in learning organizations. One could envisage the creation of a position of a 'Director of Learning': the holder of such a position would be required to undertake evaluation and change roles consistent with those discussed in this section.

REFERENCES

Alkin, M. and Dalliak, R. (1985). *A Guide for Evaluation Decision Makers*. Beverly Hills, CA: Sage.

Alkin, M. C., Daillak, R. and White, P. (1979). *Using Evaluations: Does Evaluation Make a Difference?* Sage Library of Social Research, vol. 76. Beverly Hills, CA: Sage.

Alkin, M. C. and Taut, S. M. (2003). Unbundling evaluation use. *Studies in Educational Evaluation*, 29, 1–12.

Chelimsky, E. (ed.) (1977). *A Symposium on the Use of Evaluation by Federal Agencies*, vol. 2. McLean, VA: Mitre Corporation.

Conley-Tyler, M. (2005). A fundamental choice: Internal or external evaluation? *Evaluation Journal of Australasia*, 4(1/2), 3–11.

Cousins, J. B. and Leithwood, K. A. (1986). Current empirical research on evaluation utilization. *Review of Educational Research*, 56(3), 331–364.

Downs, A. (1967). *Inside Bureaucracies*. Boston, MA: Little, Brown.

Greene, J. (1988). Stakeholder participation and utilization in program evaluation. *Evaluation Review*, 12, 91–116.

Hendricks, M. (1994). Making a splash: Reporting evaluation results effectively. In J. S. Wholey, H. P. Hatrey and K. Newcomer (eds), *Handbook of Practical Program Evaluation* (pp. 576–589). San Francisco: Jossey-Bass.

Hendricks, M. and Papagiannis, M. (1990). Do's and don'ts for offering effective recommendations. *Evaluation Practice*, 11(2), 121–125.

Henry, G. T. and Mark, M. M. (2003). Beyond use: Understanding evaluation's influence on attitudes and actions. *American Journal of Evaluation*, 24(3), 293–314.

Hudson-Mabbs, S. (1993). *Influences on the Use of Evaluation Information*. Unpublished Master of Education (Hons) thesis, Murdoch University, Perth, WA.

Johnson, R. B. (1998). Towards a theoretical model of evaluation utilization. *Evaluation and Program Planning*, 21, 93–110.

Johnston, W. P. (ed.) (1988). Increasing Evaluation Use: Some Observations Based on Results at the US General Accounting Office. *New Directions for Program Evaluation*, 39, 75–84.

Kirkhart, K. E. (2000). Reconceptualizing evaluation use: An integrated theory of influence. *New Directions for Evaluation*, 88, 5–23.

Knott, J. and Wildavsky, A. (1980). If Dissemination is the Solution, What is the Problem? *Knowledge: Creation, Diffusion, Utilization*, 1(4) (June), 537–75.

Lipton, D. S. (1992). How to maximize utilization of evaluation research by policymakers. *Annals of the American Academy of Political and Social Science*, 521(May), 175–188.

Macy, D. L. (1981). Research briefs. In N. L. Smith (ed.), *Communication Strategies in Evaluation*, Vol. 3. Beverly Hills, CA: Sage.

Mowbray, C. T. (1988). Getting the system to respond to evaluation findings. *New Directions for Program Evaluation*, 39, 21–33.

Muscatello, D. B. (ed.) (1988). Developing an Agenda that Works: The Right Choice at the Right Time. *New Directions for Program Evaluation*, 39, 21–33.

Owen, J. M. (1984). *Evaluating Teacher Education in Australia: The Use of National Guidelines in Assessing the Worth of a Program in Action.* Paper presented at the annual meeting of the American Educational Research Association, New Orleans.

Owen, J. M., Getty, C. and Simonelli, A. (1996). *Responding to the Educational Needs of Schools: Implications for the Australian Council for Educational Research* (Evaluation Report): Centre for Program Evaluation, The University of Melbourne.

Owen, J. M., Johnson, N. J. and Welsh, R. J. (1985). *Primary Concerns: A Project on Mathematics and Science in Primary Teacher Education.* Melbourne, Vic: Melbourne College of Advanced Education, for the Commonwealth Tertiary Education Commission.

Owen, J. M., Lambert, F. C. and Stringer, W. S. (1994). Acquiring knowledge of implementation and change: Essential for program evaluators? *Knowledge: Creation, Diffusion, Utilization*, 15(3), 273–294.

Owen, J. M. and Lambert, F. C. (1995). Roles for evaluation in learning organizations. *Evaluation*, 1(2), 259–273.

Owen, J. M. and McLeod, J. (1991). *A Detailed Proposal for Protective Services Training Evaluation.* Report to the Manager, Child Protection Services: Community Services Victoria.

Patton, M. Q. (1997). *Utilization Focused Evaluation*, 3rd ed. Thousand Oaks, CA: Sage.

Patton, M. Q. (2003). Utilization-focused evaluation. In K. T and D. L. Stufflebeam (eds), *International Handbook of Educational Evaluation*, vol. 9 (pp. 223–244). London: Kluwer.

Pelz, D. (1978). Some expanded perspectives on use of social science in public policy. In J. M. Yinger and S. J. Guther (eds), *Major Social Science Issues: A Multidisciplinary View* (pp. 346–357). New York: The Free Press.

Preskill, H. and Caracelli, V. J. (1996). *The Past, Present and Future Conceptions of Evaluation Use: Results from a Survey on Current Conceptions of Evaluation Use.* Paper presented at the American Evaluation Association, Atlanta, GA.

Preskill, H., S. and Torres, R. T. (2000). The learning dimension of evaluation use. *New Directions for Evaluation*, 88, 25–38.

Sharma, N. (2004). *Evaluation Recommendations: What Works?* Unpublished Master of Assessment and Evaluation Thesis, The University of Melbourne.

Smith, M. F. (1988). Evaluation utilization revisited. *New Directions for Program Evaluation*, 39, 7–20.

Sonnichsen, R. C. (1994). Evaluators as change agents. In J. S. Wholey, H. P. Hatrey and K. Newcomer (eds), *Handbook of Practical Program Evaluation* (pp. 576–589). San Francisco: Jossey Bass.

Weiss, C. H. (1999). The interface between evaluation and public policy. *Evaluation*, *5*(4), 468–486.

Weiss, C. H. and Bucuavalas, M. J. (1980). Truth tests and utility tests: Decision makers frames of reference for social science research. *American Sociological Review*, 45 (April), 302–313.

Wyatt, T., Carbines, R., Willett, J. and Robb, L. (2004). *National Evaluation of the Supported Accommodation Assistance Program. Future Directions for SAAP*. Commonwealth of Australia.

7 Managing Evaluation

In this chapter, we turn our attention to:

- how evaluations are managed;
- roles and influences of external evaluators;
- ways in which evaluators can work for and within organizations;
- roles and influences of internal evaluators; and
- costing of evaluation work.

MANAGING EVALUATION UNDERTAKEN BY OUTSIDERS

Contracting Evaluations

A common arrangement for undertaking evaluations is for a commissioning agency to contract out or outsource the work to an outsider, an evaluation consultant. Perhaps the agency does not have the expertise to undertake the study itself, or senior managers see the need for an independent group to examine a program that is to be reviewed.

A contracted evaluation can be thought of as a project, providing value for the resources that are expended. Value can be represented by the provision of findings that provide leverage in decision-making about the intervention under review.

One might expect that contracted evaluation work would always provide knowledge of value to those who commission it. But there are many examples of results that are of little or no use because the commissioning agent did not have the expertise, or did not devote the time to ensuring that the evaluation project began and remained on track.

Given this, commissioning agencies need to be clear about what they expect from evaluation studies. Well-organized agencies appoint experienced staff as evaluation managers to handle all aspects of the evaluation process, from the development of the brief to the acceptance of the final report.

Preparing a brief

While it was once the norm for commissioners to have a hazy idea of what they required from an evaluation, it is now far more likely that they will have prepared a clear brief, or Request for Proposal (RFP), before tenders are called. The development of an RFP can be thought of as a first milestone in the effective management of an evaluation. Good briefs usually come about through agency staff working through the detail of what is needed, perhaps using a content or evaluation expert to ensure that the brief is internally consistent.

Having a prepared brief provides a clear starting point for selecting an evaluator to undertake the study or studies. Potential evaluators need to know that the brief is ready, and an advertisement in the press is often used for this purpose. Some government departments keep a list of potential evaluators, and the availability of email makes the task of alerting them and sending the RFP a relatively easy and inexpensive exercise.

Depending on the nature and scope of the evaluation, briefs vary in complexity. A recent example from one government agency contained the following sections:

1 statement of requirements;
2 evaluation methodology;
3 conditions of tendering;
4 schedules;
5 confidentiality clauses;
6 government requirements; and
7 declaration by the tenderer.

Of these sections, only the first two relate to the evaluation plan for the study; the others outline legal arrangements seeking assurance that the consultant is bona fide. In this particular case, the brief provided a minimal amount of information about what was actually required by the evaluation audience.

A more extensive and balanced brief would contain the following:

- purposes of the evaluation;
- background and context for the study;
- key questions and the kinds of knowledge products required (for example, recommendations);

- number and nature of reports;
- criteria for tender selection;
- time frame;
- proposal deadline;
- an indication of the expected cost range; and
- legal requirements, including the bona fides of the tenderer.

For large studies, agencies should proffer a briefing session which allows potential tenderers to ask questions and seek points of clarification before submitting their proposal.

Agencies usually assemble a steering committee to manage an evaluation project. While this is best set up at the very beginning, at the time a decision is made to undertake the project, most steering committees are formed at about the time the brief is distributed.

Steering committees are a way of catering for a wide range of stakeholders in the program being evaluated; sometimes, because of their size, they can become unwieldy in terms of managing the evaluation study. One solution is to set up an advisory committee to handle evaluation management matters on a day-to-day basis.

Example 7.1 Managing a complex national level evaluation

A Coordination and Development Committee (CAD) commissioned evaluations of a national Supported Accommodation Assistance Scheme (SAAP). The CAD represented parties responsible, including the state and federal government, for the provision of housing to the homeless. In evaluations undertaken in 1998 and 2003, the CAD created the position of Evaluation Manager, a senior departmental officer, and set up a technical reference group (TRG) for the duration of each study. The TRG was made up of representatives from the CAD and co-opted members with expertise in homelessness and evaluation. The TRG developed an evaluation brief, set up procedures to select the consultant, liaised with the consultant about the evaluation design, received and commented upon draft reports, and met with the CAD when the report was in the penultimate stage. TRG members attended sessions during which data were collected from group respondents, and the evaluation manager kept in touch with the principals of the consultancy group throughout the study.

All stakeholders viewed the TRG as an 'honest broker' between the CAD and the evaluation consultants. Initially conceived as a committee that would concentrate on methodology, the TRG expanded its responsibilities considerably to become involved in the evaluation process more generally. The CAD has been favorably disposed to these processes, which are seen to be innovatory by some evaluation theorists (Wyatt et al. 2004).

Selection of an evaluation consultant is itself an evaluative activity. A steering committee should set up a rigorous process that can withstand any request under freedom of information regulations, if they apply.

Example 7.2 Choosing the evaluation consultant

To choose a consultant for a large-scale evaluation, one member of the evaluation steering committee developed a 'selection grid'. The grid was in the form of a matrix which contained the criteria listed in the brief on one axis and the names of all applicants on the other. Each criterion was given a weighting that had been previously agreed upon, and had been indicated in the RFP. Steering committee members were asked, independently, to rate each proposal on all criteria. Each member then brought these ratings to a meeting of committee members. Scores for each consultant were determined by averaging the scores of each member, taking into account the weightings. This led to the ranking of the applications and the selection of the consultant for the project.

Hawkins (2003) provides examples of criteria that can be used, as follows:

- contractor's track record;
- adequacy of response to the RFP;
- quality of the methodology (to answer the evaluation questions);
- implementation details;
- communication and reporting strategies;
- competencies of the consultancy team; and
- value for money.

Preparing an evaluation proposal

The most important aspect of a proposal is an evaluation plan, as discussed in Chapter 4. Development of the proposal itself is a management task for leaders of consultancy teams and is usually handled by senior members of these teams. In general terms, a decision to respond to an RFP should be made with full knowledge of other commitments the team has, or is likely to have, over the period during which the study must be undertaken. There is a tendency for consultancy teams to over-commit and under-resource their studies—in other words, to promise commissioners more than they can provide in an effort to secure the contract. In some cases, expertise and experience may be confined to one only or two staff, who are thus stretched thinly across many commitments. Inexperienced and part-time staff are employed to fill in the gaps, and the final report disappoints the commissioners, leaving bad tastes in the mouths all-round. A warning sign that this scenario will eventuate is the listing in an evaluation proposal of several senior staff who will spend very small proportions of their 'billable time', less than a day a week, on a given study. Effective evaluation work almost always requires the continuous presence of a senior experienced evaluator during most, if not all, of the period of a study.

Sometimes contracting agencies invoke a two-stage model of proposal development. In the first stage, potential evaluators are asked to provide a brief expression of interest. On this basis, a small number of applicants is asked to prepare a comprehensive proposal. This reduces the preparatory work required of consultants, and is seen as a positive step because of savings in time and energy for all concerned (Jakob-Hoff 2003).

Managing the study after selecting a consultant

Until recently, it was customary for the selected evaluator to 'go away' and undertake the investigation, reporting back to the steering committee at the end of the investigation. Now, however, steering committees tend to interact more intensively with their consultant throughout the entire evaluation process. These committees often incorporate evaluation expertise, have more say in decisions about the evaluation design and demand greater justification for the methods that evaluators plan to use. An experienced commissioner of evaluations provides this point of view:

> A high-quality evaluation is more likely to be achieved if the purchaser and the contractor work together. It is not sufficient to leave the contractor to get on with the work and wait for him or her to deliver the milestone reports. Development of a good working relationship, with regular communication, is essential. Given the complex and technical nature of evaluation, active management is required to prevent the evaluation going off the rails (Hawkins 2003, p. 55).

An experienced consultant provides this point of view:

> Relationships between purchasers and contractors are of critical importance in successful contracting. An effective relationship needs to exist between the two parties to allow for effective resolution of problems as and when they arise—and they always arise. The fact is, most problems in evaluations cannot be dealt with in service contracts, and other means, based on good working relationships, must be used.
>
> A good working relationship is also needed to ensure that the results can be used to their fullest extent. A contractor cannot guarantee this without the assistance of purchaser staff (Jakob-Hoff 2003, p. 59).

These working relationships must be designed to ensure that the implementation of the evaluation project proceeds smoothly. Generally the commissioner takes the running on key matters such as asking for and receiving interim reports, negotiating changes of emphases in evaluation direction, receiving draft reports and providing feedback to the writers, disseminating findings to stakeholders, and authorizing payments to the evaluators. In the exercise of these matters a balance must be struck between the independence of the evaluation team and the need for the study to stay focused to meet the agenda that initiated the evaluation project.

GUIDELINES FOR EVALUATION BY OUTSIDERS

As we have just seen, many agencies place a reliance on outsiders to undertake evaluation or provide advice on how to conduct evaluations. Outsider consulting is undertaken by:

- business management consultants;
- university departments and centers devoted to research and evaluation in a range of disciplines (public policy, health, social work); and
- independent one- or two-person agencies.

Scriven (1995) has some advice aimed particularly at those in the last of these categories, the small-scale or solo consultant. He believes that these consultants have a hard time making their business viable because of the competition for work from those in the other categories, in particular university departments and centers, which are effectively subsidized to do external consulting work by their institutions. Solo consultants need to acknowledge that they must attend to the following tasks:

- managing their companies on a day-to-day basis;
- making and extending contacts;

- undertaking evaluative studies;
- maintaining and extending a repertoire of evaluation skills; and
- contributing to research on evaluation.

Scriven calculates that the consultant can really only expect to spend half of a 'working year' on undertaking evaluative studies. If we take a working year to be 2,000 hours (50 weeks by 40 hours per week), this leaves 1,000 hours to actually work on evaluation studies. He reckons that a one-person consultant without a secretary and working from a home office would need to gross $55,000 to clear $40,000, given overheads, company costs and other expenses, including indemnity insurance. This means charging $55 per hour, or about $500 per day. Scriven also makes the point that the effective solo practitioner has to be good at finding and maintaining contacts, which he refers to as 'hustling' for jobs. This has little to do with the skills normally associated with evaluation work. Individuals who move from paid employment to consulting often do not make it as a solo consultant because they are unable or unwilling to put in the sustained effort to bring in a steady stream of work.

All consultants need to keep an eye out for evaluation projects and be in a position to tender successfully for those they find attractive. This requires the consultant to manage all stages of the tendering process outlined at the beginning of this chapter.

Costs of evaluation studies

The costs of an evaluation study will obviously vary according to the scope of the work done—however, there are obviously limits on the resources that should be spent on a given study. For example, it would be ludicrous for the evaluation of a program to exceed the cost of the program itself. When pressed to provide a 'ballpark' figure by those planning to build in evaluation from the beginning of a program—an admirable strategy—we suggest a figure of 10–15 percent.

The tender submission should always include a statement of the budget based on the cost of personnel, travel and overheads. The following is a hypothetical example based on an actual evaluation of a major educational policy.

Example 7.3 Budget for the evaluation of a major educational policy

The evaluation plan requires that evaluators spend extensive periods of time in eighteen case study schools. Non-participant observation will be the approach used. This includes the use of interviews, observation of key events and meetings, and examination of documents at each site. It will be necessary to visit each site regularly during the school year. Staff with knowledge of schools and an ability to collect and understand the data will be needed.

As indicated in an earlier part of the plan, the study needs to be coordinated so that there are common methodological approaches in both the collection and analysis phases. This will require an evaluation director with these skills.

It will be necessary for one full-time field worker to be employed for the duration of the study, a period of twelve months, supported by the director of the consulting firm.

Costing

- *Evaluation Staff*. Salary of one field coordinator $65,000 plus 30 percent on-costs for 52 weeks:
  $84,500
- *Evaluation Director*. The study will require a director who will be responsible for coordination of the evaluation and the development of the data management approach. The director will be involved for one day a week for 40 weeks (0.8 year at 0.2 time) during the year at an annual salary of ($85,000 x 0.2 x 0.8) plus 30 percent overheads:
  $17,680
- *Administrative/Secretarial*. On the basis of one day per week for 40 weeks (0.8 time). Salary ($35,000 x 0.2 x 0.8) plus 30 percent overheads:
  $7,280
- *Travel*. On the basis of 30 days accommodation and car hire @ $250 per day, plus miscellaneous metropolitan travel ($500):
  $8,000
- Printing of report and distribution:
  $500
- Miscellaneous (computer analyses, telephone, etc.):
  $1,000
- Total:
  $118,960
- Add organizational on costs @ 30 percent:
  $35,690

Grand total:
$154,380

It can be seen here that the consulting firm built in a 30 percent overhead cost to allow for the 'other tasks' that consultants need to do, as indicated earlier by Scriven. As an alternative to setting out details of salaries and other costs, some larger consulting firms calculate a daily cost of an employee for consulting. This varies according to several factors, including the base salary of the employee. Rates for a highly regarded evaluation consultant can go as high as $3,000 per day. While some consultants have fixed rates, others vary their charges according to what the market can bear. Some university-based evaluation centers adopt a sliding scale of rates according to the client, charging less for work done where the client may have very limited resources.

Outsider for insider evaluations

These are situations where an external evaluator is asked to review a program for an internal audience. This arrangement is predicated on the need for special expertise and a requirement for an 'objective' view of the program under review.

Example 7.4 Evaluation of a human development program

Hurworth et al. (1988) undertook an evaluation of a program designed to educate 15–16-year-olds about issues relating to contraception, sexually transmitted diseases and the dangers of drug abuse.

The major reason for the evaluation was to establish program worth before a decision was made to promote it for adoption by other health centers across the state. The clients saw a need for an external evaluator to add credibility to the findings.

The design of the evaluation was decided upon through consultancy with the clients, the providers of the program (two nurses and a doctor), and included a strong outcomes emphasis. The findings showed that the program promoted learning and was well regarded by students and their teachers.

The evaluators reported to the clients and to the administration of the health center through a written report. A seminar which was attended by key health care decision-makers was also part of the reporting process.

There is sometimes a perception of threat from the presence of an outsider. Thus outside evaluators working within this arrangement should become familiar with the needs of the internal audiences and ensure that the evaluation is responsive to the needs of the agency. Experience suggests that the more the evaluator can work with the insiders from the outset of an evaluation, the more clients will come to trust the evaluator and use the findings to make changes suggested by the evaluation (Owen 1990).

Outsider for insider evaluations can be used by senior management to legitimate downsizing organizations under their control. In some cases unscrupulous managers have used external reviewers—generally highly paid business management consultants—to help them with 'hatchet jobs' that have led to staff layoffs or considerable reductions in organizational operations. The term 'unscrupulous' can be applied particularly to managers who have already decided that layoffs are to take place, and subsequently influence the organizational review to provide findings which are consistent with decisions that have already been made. This has occurred not only in the private sector, but is also evident in government and higher education sectors. Such reviews could not be regarded as evaluation, as the consultant's work is unlikely to meet the codes of behavior set by the evaluation profession as discussed in Chapter 8.

Outsider for outsider evaluations

In these situations there is a sense of an evaluation 'done on' a program. The expertise and objectivity of the evaluation team is valued by the evaluation commissioners. Program providers are not involved in the planning of the evaluation; they are expected to provide information but are unlikely to benefit directly in terms of feedback of information or support to improve their work. Evaluation findings are targeted to a 'higher authority'.

Example 7.5 Evaluation of the Participation and Equity Program (PEP)

The Participation and Equity Program (PEP) was the linchpin of a national education strategy for reform of secondary schools and community colleges. PEP was a three-year intervention but, despite its scope and importance, no monitoring procedures had been built into the finding for the initiative.

Owen and Hartley (1988) undertook an analysis of the impact of the national PEP program on community colleges. Insiders in this case were the colleges which were recipients of assistance to enable them to develop programs for educationally disadvantaged young people.

The analysis involved a state-by-state review of systemic responses to the PEP initiative, and a series of case studies of specific examples of the implementation of programs supported by PEP. Findings were presented in an extensive report and a volume of case studies. The primary audience was officers in the government department which was responsible for the PEP initiative, and it was to these officers that the report was presented.

Under these circumstances, it is understandable that the staff responsible for the delivery of the program might find excuses for non-cooperation, especially if the findings could be potentially damaging to them in one way or another. Nevertheless, we have found people from a range of social program areas willing to assist in large-scale outsider for outsider studies. In many cases the motivation is altruistic. In practice, this facilitates the compilation of information, which assists decision-makers, generally policy-makers, to make decisions about existing social programs.

GUIDELINES FOR EVALUATION BY INSIDERS

Insider for insider evaluations

These are situations where the evaluator and provider are employed by the agency responsible for the program. Evaluation is 'in-house', findings of the study may not be made available to the general public, and may be informally presented to key decision-makers. Sometimes internal evaluations adopting this configuration are referred to as *institutional self-study*.

The focus in this arrangement is generally on organizational learning and program improvement. This approach to evaluation relies for its validity on the availability of internal expertise. This implies that agencies see benefits in providing human and material resources for evaluation support for programs.

The insiders for insiders arrangement manifests itself in various ways. Generally it requires an agency to adopt a commitment to the accumulation of knowledge about itself—that is, it adopts a continuous learning focus (Morris 1995). This includes the generation and documentation of new knowledge on the services it provides to clients, experiences about individual programs that might be extrapolated to other like situations, and on the internal work climate of the organization itself (Torres et al. 1996). The primary audience could be delivery staff or management.

A commitment to insider for insider evaluations is well established in some school systems in the United States (Alkin 1990) and is emerging in countries such as Japan. Research across these and other countries has found that teachers usually take on evaluation as an addition to day-to-day administrative and classroom tasks. In practice, teachers have sometimes been asked to undertake evaluation work without the benefit of training. That evaluation is often treated as an 'extra' on top of a normal teaching load, leads to frustration and cynicism about the benefits that evaluation can provide. Insider-for-insider evaluation can exhaust participants but, when well resourced, can have a powerful impact on the staff and programs of a school (Brennan & Hoadley 1984).

Experience suggests that evaluation undertaken in this configuration can be extremely useful for within-organization decision-making if adequate person-centered resources are made available. In the United States, the National Education Association's Mastery in Schools project was a case where a small number of schools were supported by an external evaluation and development consultant who, to all intents and purposes, became an additional staff member of the school (Holly 1990).

Generally, insider-for-insider evaluations tend to use Approaches consistent with the Clarificative and Interactive evaluation Forms, although recently there has been a greater expectation, at least in the United States, that organizations will document program outcomes (Hatry & van Houten 1996).

It is important to note that an evaluator can act as an insider without necessarily being employed by the agency commissioning the evaluation. The key is that the evaluator acts as a 'psychological' insider—that is, he or she is in tune with the agency and is willing to provide evaluative advice designed to improve its functions. This does not mean that the evaluator provides only findings that the primary audience wants to hear. The ideal situation is that clients genuinely want information, which they may find both positive and negative, which will be used to make their programs more effective. Our experience working in this mold is that many organizations committed to learning about themselves are keen to employ 'critical friends' who are fearless in giving advice and, when the occasion is right, will extend a helping hand to assist with implementing changes that flow from the evaluation (Telford 1991).

Cummings (1988) and others see the following advantages of insider evaluators:

- They reduce evaluation costs.
- They are in a position to alter evaluation designs quickly if it becomes apparent that an evaluation activity is not productive.
- They know the nuances of the agency and are thus able to see ways in which an evaluation can make a difference.
- They can build a strong credibility over time and can foster stakeholder commitment and promote the use of evaluation findings.

On the other hand:

- Their objectivity may be affected or compromised by the policies of the organization and its underlying value system.
- They could become a public relations tool of the organization to the detriment of other more legitimate roles such as encouraging program improvement.

Internal evaluation and change

Organizational decision-makers are increasingly looking for assistance with process re-engineering and people-related facets of change management. The distinction between organizational development consultants and evaluators is becoming blurred. Often an organizational development consultant will be brought in to accomplish a range of tasks, including diagnosing organizational culture, working with the staff to identify change initiatives and undertaking a training needs analysis. These tasks fall within the domain and skill set traditionally associated with the practice of evaluation and could be handled by a skilled internal evaluator.

Mathison (1994) suggests that a critical distinction that separates evaluation from organizational development is the separation of evaluative judgment and prescription. She claims that evaluators are ill equipped to provide recommendations because these require much greater knowledge than can be subsumed by the evaluation study itself. However, increasingly, there is an opportunity for evaluators to adopt a participatory framework for conducting evaluations—one that recognizes the importance of involving program stakeholders in the evaluation process. Such collaborative arrangements clear the way for the creation of prescriptions involving evaluator and stakeholders. We have documented the advantages of internal and external evaluators working in such a mode:

> We believe that an evaluator with requisite skills and knowledge is in a unique position to assist stakeholders to maximize the instrumental use of the findings. It is the evaluator who has worked with the

> organization over a period of time through the various states of negotiation, data collection, and reporting back. Given sound human relations skills, the evaluator has the opportunity to build a strong sense of trust and a high level of rapport with those within the organization, and to develop a shared understanding of the meaning and the implications of the assembled information. With a high personal stake in the quality of the study, the evaluator is then in a position to encourage an informed and balanced use of the findings (Owen et al. 1994).

There is a clear role for evaluators to work directly with those in leadership positions. It is not necessarily always the case that those in formal positions of responsibility will be the leaders in the organizational change or program improvement effort.

Some of the more radical aspects that an internal evaluator could focus on include: surfacing and challenging assumptions, analyzing organizational culture, assisting with strategic thinking and planning, and promoting learning within the organization. These issues have been identified from the organizational literature as key to the success of a learning organization (Owen & Lambert 1998).

While some evaluators may be uneasy about adopting a strongly developmental role, the reality is that organizational development consultants are already working in these ways without the benefit of extensive training in evaluation design or data analytical methods, or a well-developed underlying epistemological basis. With more and more evaluative work being nested in agencies (Love 1994), there should be increasing opportunities for those with strong analytical and communication skills to play an influential role in key decision-making. As with all hard-nosed business decisions, a judgment about the advantages of employing an internal evaluator will depend on whether those who control the purse strings see a pay-off for the evaluative services provided.

Insider for outsider evaluations

These situations also involve self-evaluation, but in this arrangement the findings are addressed to an outside audience or audiences. A typical scenario for this kind of evaluation is one in which an agency has obtained external funding for an internally designed program. A condition is that insiders must report to the funders, setting out the benefits that have accrued as a result of program implementation. There is usually an emphasis on program outcomes, consistent with the tenets of the Impact evaluation Form.

One issue related to this configuration of evaluation is the validity of evaluation findings. Continued funding of programs may be dependent on these findings, and in such circumstances it would be a brave organization that placed a heavy emphasis on negative aspects of program impact. A negative report may also have implications for program directors and reduce the chance that funding will be granted for other projects. It is up to the primary audience in this case to be aware that program development and implementation involve risk-taking and that a balance in reporting involving positive and negative outcomes is to be expected. In fact, an enlightened funding body should become suspicious of an evaluation report that is entirely positive.

An example of the use of this configuration is accreditation. Hospitals, nursing and aged care institutions, and universities are typical subjects of accreditation procedures. An end-product of an accreditation is a plan of action for the next period of program delivery—for example, five years. The report to outsiders is in the form of a justification for the evaluation procedures undertaken and the decisions about the future, should accreditation be granted.

In the case of accreditation, the problem of validation of the information collected by insiders is solved by reference to externally developed procedures and the use of visiting expert panels. Sometimes, system-wide standards are used in conjunction with the internal evaluation. This is designed to prove that the programs within a hospital or a university have credibility in the eyes of the general public, and in particular to prospective clients (patients, students) of the program.

An in-principle organizational commitment to internal evaluation implies that managers foresee a net benefit in providing resources for internal evaluative work. To keep faith with management, internal evaluators need to understand how to operate within a framework that acknowledges the hierarchy, and the internal structure and culture of the organization.

A review of practice suggests that internal evaluations are more effective if the administration accepts the following principles:

- Involve the staff, or those staff directly engaged in the delivery of the program under review, as much as possible in the planning and implementation of each study. The more staff contribute to evaluation decisions, the more enthusiastic they will be. Meetings at which staff are given an opportunity to understand concepts and ideas, and the advantages of self-evaluation, can be very useful.
- A group responsible for the day-to-day management of the evaluation should be formed. This might include staff with limited evaluation expertise in addition to the internal evaluator. During the evaluation planning stage, specify the responsibilities and limitations of the group—for example, collecting and analyzing data, but not drawing conclusions.

- Ensure that there is consensus, or almost consensus, on the evaluation plan, even if this appears to take a large amount of time and effort. Make sure that the agency leadership is aware of the details.
- Ensure that the evaluation team has the necessary resources for the collection and analysis of the data. This may involve technical advice from the internal evaluator or an outside expert on data collection and analysis at some stage. If the evaluation is concerned with Monitoring, establish an ongoing record-keeping system. Develop procedures which ensure that the data can be entered into the system at regular intervals.
- Encourage the evaluators to report on their progress even if they are not in a position to report on their findings.
- Use the findings to reflect on the program or agency aspects under review. Decide on the changes that should be made and to what—for example, whether implementation processes should be modified so that objectives can be achieved.
- Develop a systematic plan by which program changes can be put in place. Changing the program can be difficult, but it is most important in improving the program and benefiting those served by it.

REFERENCES

Alkin, M. C. (1990). *Debates on Evaluation.* Newbury Park, CA: Sage.

Brennan, M. and Hoadley, R. (1984). *School Self Evaluation.* Melbourne: Education Department of Victoria.

Cummings, O. W. (1988). Business perspectives on internal/external evaluation. *New Directions for Program Evaluation*, 39, 59–74.

Hatry, H. P. and van Houten, T. (1996). *Measuring Program Outcomes.* Washington, DC: United Way of America.

Hawkins, P. (2003). Contracting evaluation: A tender topic. In N. Lunt, C. Davidson and K. McKegg (eds), *Evaluating Policy and Practice: A New Zealand Reader* (pp. 48–57). Auckland, NZ: Pearson Education New Zealand Ltd.

Holly, P. (1990). *Growth from Within: A New Paradigm for Educational Evaluation.* Paper held at the Centre for Program Evaluation, The University of Melbourne.

Hurworth, R. E., Owen J. M. and Griffin, L. D. (1988). *The Impact of the Richmond Community Health Centre Pre-Pregnancy Program.* Melbourne: Centre for Program Evaluation, The University of Melbourne.

Jakob-Hoff, M. (2003). A provider perspective of current practice in the commissioning of evaluation in New Zealand. In N. Lunt, C. Davidson and K. McKegg (eds), *Evaluating Policy and Practice: A New Zealand Reader* (pp. 58–63). Auckland, NZ: Pearson Education New Zealand Ltd.

Love, A. (1994). Internal evaluation: Building organizations from within. In *International Conference of the Australasian Evaluation Society*. Canberra: Australasian Evaluation Society.

Mathison, S. (1994). Rethinking the evaluation role: Partnerships between organizations and evaluators. *Evaluation and Program Planning*, 17(3), 299–304.

Morris, L. E. (1995). Developing strategies for the knowledge era. In S. Chawla and J. Renesch, (eds), *Learning Organizations*. Portland, OR: Productivity Press.

Owen, J. M. (1990). Encouraging small-scale evaluation: Roles for an external evaluator. *Evaluation Journal of Australasia*, 2(3), 41–50.

Owen, J. M. and Hartley, R. (1988). *Case Studies in Five TAFE Colleges*. Melbourne: Department of Employment, Education and Training.

Owen, J. M. and Lambert, F. C. (1998). Evaluation and the information needs of organizational leaders. *American Journal of Evaluation*, 19, (3), 355–365.

Owen, J. M., Lambert, F. C. and Stringer, W. S. (1994). Acquiring knowledge of implementation and change: Essential for program evaluators? *Knowledge: Creation, Diffusion, Utilization*, 15(3), 273–294.

Scriven, M. (1995). Evaluation consulting. *Evaluation Practice*, 16(1), 47–57.

Telford, H. (1991). *Responsive Evaluation for Development in Self Managing Schools*. Unpublished paper for the degree of Doctor of Education, The University of Melbourne.

Torres, R. T., Preskill, H. S. and Piontek, M. E. (1996). *Evaluation Strategies for Communicating and Reporting: Enhancing Learning Organizations*. Thousand Oaks, CA: Sage.

Wyatt, T., Carbines, R., Willett, J. and Robb, L. (2004). *National Evaluation of the Supported Accommodation Assistance Program (SAAP IV)*. Canberra: Commonwealth of Australia.

Codes of Behavior for Evaluators

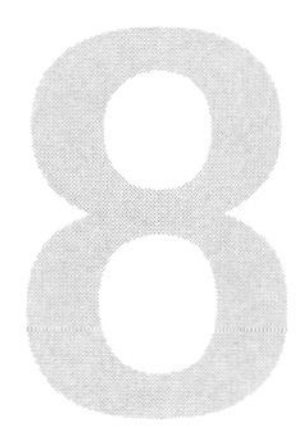

In this chapter we examine codes of behavior that should be applied to evaluative inquiry. These guidelines are predicated on a belief that evaluators, stakeholders and others should have reference points from which to judge whether evaluation practice is acceptable. We have mentioned these codes in passing earlier, in Chapter 4. Here they are described and discussed in more detail.

CODES OF BEHAVIOR FOR APPLIED SOCIAL SCIENCE RESEARCH

Among agencies and professions which support social science research, there has long been concern that the procedures and methods used take into account the rights and welfare of participants (Homan 1991). For example, the informed consent of participants is commonly required for all research undertaken by universities and allied institutions. Informed consent is a procedure by which individuals choose whether or not to participate in a study after being presented with information that impinges on this decision. Ethics committees rigorously review all research designs developed by university faculty. Issues that these committees consider include:

- the rationale and need for the study;
- the quality of the design;
- whether a competent and qualified practitioner supervises the research;
- adequacy of material support; and
- appropriate selection of participants or groups.

In some instances, there must be assurances that adequate reparations can be made to those who may be disadvantaged by publications of the findings of the study.

When professionals with accredited credentials undertake research, they are expected to abide by the code of behavior of their professional body. Associations such as the American Anthropological Association have developed codes of behavior, and members are expected to become acquainted with them as part of their induction. Agencies such as the US Accounting Office have similar codes for staff working on audits conducted by the Office. Codes of behavior generally consist of a set of standards of practice. Each standard can be regarded as a principle mutually agreed to by people engaged in a given profession—a principle that, if met, enhances the fairness and quality of that practice.

The existence of professional standards can present moral dilemmas for the researcher working within or for an organization. This is almost always the case for evaluators. In such contexts, the investigator may take a position that will lead to conflict. For example, the investigator might not agree with the goals of a given programmatic intervention, or be at odds with the ways in which management has implemented the program. In an analysis of such relationships, Mirvis and Seashore (1982) concluded that the very nature of an organizational system necessitates that researchers approach participants and ethical issues differently from those in non-applied settings—for example, in laboratory experiments. In organizational settings, participants in research cannot be approached as individuals without management first being contacted. This is because of the hierarchical and interdependent nature of roles and relationships in such organizations.

Within an organizational situation, researchers do not have the power to resolve all ethical dilemmas—for example, to ensure the well-being of participants, or to make assurances that the research will be carried out as planned. This conclusion led Mirvis and Seashore to suggest that researchers need to modify their approach to behavioral codes in such settings by moving from applying prescriptive guidelines and standards to using these more flexibly, according to the situation at hand. Having reached what might be regarded as a realistic position, it is up to the researcher to communicate these expectations to stakeholders and clients. In summary, it is the researcher's responsibility as ethical decision-maker 'to create roles that are mutually clarified and compatible, and, in creating them, to affirm general ethical norms governing human research' (Mirvis & Seashore 1982).

The researcher and the organization need to reach agreement on the ethical principles that underlie an investigation. An implication is that, if such agreement cannot be reached early in the study, the researcher might consider withdrawing from the situation.

CODES OF BEHAVIOR FOR EVALUATION

Evaluative inquiry is a branch of applied social science research. Thus the discussion in the previous section is relevant to most evaluations. Many of these issues will be familiar to those who have undertaken evaluation, even if they have not been aware of relevant formalized codes of behavior. For example, the evaluator needs to honor promises of anonymity and confidentiality. Evaluation designs that involve control groups need to be carefully examined for potential ethical risks. Reporting ought to include fair attention to the strengths and weaknesses of programs.

Evaluation is always conducted within the context of the needs of individuals or organizations, be they from the helping professions, government or private agencies. The evaluator can be regarded as an outsider or insider relative to the client, and the evaluative contribution might include that of consultant, educator or change agent. These roles can lead to conflict between the evaluator and management, or between evaluator and program provider. The reputation and career of the evaluator depend on providing accurate and fearless information, while a program manager's career is likely to be bound up with the provision of successful programs: 'speaking truth is a risky and painful task, but this is what the evaluator has to do' (Chelimsky 1995).

Over the past decade, the development of codes of behavior or practice has become a major issue for the evaluation profession. Guidelines have been developed in countries where there is a well-established evaluation society, such as the United States and Canada. The Australasian Evaluation Society produced its Guidelines for the Ethical Conduct of Evaluations in early 1998 and their use has been strongly supported by influential members of the society (Fraser 2001). However, the most comprehensive effort on codes of behavior has been made in the United States. These appear in the form of Program Evaluation Standards and Guiding Principles for Evaluators, each of which is now discussed in turn.

THE PROGRAM EVALUATION STANDARDS

The Program Evaluation Standards are the result of the work of the Joint Committee on Standards for Educational Evaluation. The Committee was created in 1975 with a brief to develop standards for educational evaluation after earlier work had been done on standards in test construction and administration. Major products have been the Standards for Evaluation of Educational Programs, Projects, and Materials (1981), Personnel Evaluation Standards (1988), Program

Evaluation Standards (1994) and the Student Evaluation Standards (2003). The Joint Committee is sponsored by fifteen organizations, including the American Evaluation Association. The operating procedures of the Committee were accredited by the American National Standards Institute (ANSI) in 1995, which subsequently approved the Program Evaluation Standards in 1994 (Sanders 1994).

There are 30 Program Evaluation Standards grouped within four clusters:

- utility;
- feasibility;
- propriety; and
- accuracy.

They are formalized in extensive documentation that provides an overview of each standard, case studies showing how they can be used, and how they might be violated. The characteristics of the standards are outlined below.

- *Utility standards* are intended to help in the planning of evaluations that are informative, timely and influential. Utility standards are concerned with whether an evaluation provides practical information needs for a given audience. The utility standards are listed below.

  U1 Stakeholder Identification
  Persons involved in or affected by the evaluation should be identified so that their needs can be addressed.

  U2 Evaluator Credibility
  The persons conducting the evaluation should be both trustworthy and competent to perform the evaluation, so that their findings achieve maximum credibility and acceptance.

  U3 Information Scope and Selection
  Information collected should be broadly selected to address pertinent questions about the program and be responsive to the needs and interests of clients and other specified stakeholders.

  U4 Valuation Interpretation
  The perspectives, procedures and rationale used to interpret the findings should be carefully described, so that the bases for value judgments are clear.

  U5 Report Clarity
  Evaluation reports should clearly describe the program being evaluated, including its context, and the purposes, procedures, and findings of the evaluation, so that essential information is provided and easily understood.

U6 Report Timeliness and Dissemination
Significant interim findings and evaluation reports should be disseminated to intended users, so that they can be used in a timely fashion.

U7 Evaluation Impact
Evaluations should be planned and conducted and reported in ways that encourage follow-through by stakeholders, so that the likelihood that the evaluation will be used is increased.

- *Feasibility standards* recognize that evaluations are generally conducted in natural settings. Feasibility deals with value for cost, practical issues such as availability of data, and political issues such as impact of findings. Feasibility standards call for evaluations to be realistic, diplomatic and financially well managed. The feasibility standards are listed below.

F1 Practical Procedures
The evaluation procedures should be practical, to keep disruption to a minimum, while needed information is obtained.

F2 Political Viability
The evaluation should be planned and conducted with anticipation of the different positions of various interest groups, so that their cooperation can be obtained, and so that possible attempts by any of these groups to curtail evaluation operations or to bias or misapply the results can be averted or counteracted.

F3 Cost Effectiveness
The evaluation should be efficient and produce information of sufficient value so that the resources expended can be justified.

- *Propriety standards* relate strongly to ethics. They are aimed at ensuring that the rights of people influenced by the program and its evaluation will be protected. Propriety standards require an evaluation to take into account legal and ethical issues, including the welfare of program participants and those affected by evaluation results. Proprietary standards are listed below.

P1 Service Orientation
Evaluations should be designed to assist organizations to address and effectively serve the needs of the full range of targeted participants.

P2 Formal Agreements
Obligations of the formal parties to an evaluation (what is to be done, how, and by whom, when) should be agreed to in writing, so that these parties are obliged to adhere to all conditions of the agreement or formally to renegotiate it.

P3 Rights of Human Subjects
Evaluations should be designed and conducted to respect and protect the rights and welfare of human subjects.

P4 Human Interaction
Evaluators should respect human dignity and worth in their interactions with other persons associated with an evaluation, so that participants are not threatened or harmed.

P5 Complete and Fair Assessment
The evaluation should be complete and fair in its examination and recording of strengths and weaknesses of the program being evaluated, so that strengths can be built on and problem areas addressed.

P6 Disclosure of Findings
The formal parties to an evaluation should ensure that the full set of evaluation findings along with pertinent limitations are made accessible to the persons affected by the evaluation, and any others with expressed legal rights to receive the results.

P7 Conflict of Interest
Conflict of interest should be dealt with openly and honestly, so that it does not compromise the evaluation processes and results.

P8 Fiscal Responsibility
The evaluator's allocation and expenditure of resources should reflect sound accountability procedures and otherwise be prudent and ethically responsible, so that expenditures are accounted for and appropriate.

- *Accuracy standards* determine whether an evaluation has produced truth, whether the data management reflects the key evaluation issues, whether the information is technically adequate, and that the conclusions and recommendations (if any) reflect the analysis of the data. The overall accuracy of an evaluation against these standards indicates whether the evaluation has produced valid and reliable knowledge about the program. Accuracy standards are listed below.

A1 Program Documentation
The program being evaluated should be described and documented clearly and accurately, so that the program is clearly identified.

A2 Context Analysis
The context in which the program exists should be examined in detail, so that its likely influence on the program can be identified.

A3 Described Purposes and Procedures
The purposes and procedures of the evaluation should be monitored and described in enough detail, so that they can be identified and assessed.

A4 Defensible Information Sources
The sources of information used in an evaluation should be described in enough detail, so that the adequacy of the information can be assessed.

A5 Valid Information
The information gathering procedures should be chosen or developed so that they will assure that the interpretation arrived at is valid for the intended use.

A6 Reliable Information
The information gathering procedures should be chosen or developed and then implemented so that they will assure that the information obtained is sufficiently reliable for the intended use.

A7 Systematic Information
The information collected, processed, and reported in an evaluation should be systematically reviewed and any errors found should be corrected.

A8 Analysis of Quantitative Information
Quantitative information in an evaluation should be appropriately and systematically analyzed so that the evaluation questions are effectively answered.

A9 Analysis of Qualitative Information
Qualitative information in an evaluation should be appropriately and systematically analyzed so that the evaluation questions are effectively answered.

A10 Justified Conclusions
The conclusions reached in an evaluation should be explicitly justified, so that audiences can assess them.

A11 Impartial Reporting
Reporting procedures should guard against distortion caused by personal feelings and biases to any party to the evaluation, so that evaluation reports fairly reflect the evaluation findings.

A12 Metaevaluation
The evaluation itself should be formatively and summatively evaluated against these and other pertinent standards, so that its conduct is appropriately guided and, on completion, stakeholders can closely examine its strengths and weaknesses.

GUIDING PRINCIPLES FOR EVALUATORS

The Guiding Principles for Evaluators were developed by a task force of the American Evaluation Association, and approved by a vote of the membership in 1994 (Shadish et al. 1995). The five principles and their elaboration are as follows:

Systematic inquiry
Evaluators conduct systematic, databased inquiries about whatever is being evaluated.

1 Evaluators should adhere to the highest appropriate technical standards in conjunction with their work, whether that work is quantitative or qualitative in nature, so as to increase the accuracy and credibility of the evaluative information they produce.

2 Evaluators should explore with the client the shortcomings and strengths both of the various evaluation questions it might be productive to ask, and the various approaches that might be used for answering these questions.

3 When presenting their work, evaluators should communicate their methods and approaches accurately and in sufficient detail to allow others to understand, interpret and critique their work. They should make clear the limitations of an evaluation and its results. Evaluators should discuss in a contextually appropriate way, those values, assumptions, theories, methods, results and analyses that *significantly* affect the interpretation of the evaluative findings.

These statements apply to all aspects of the evaluation, from its initial conceptualization to the eventual use of the findings.

Competence
Evaluators provide competent performance to stakeholders.

1 Evaluators should possess (or, here and elsewhere as appropriate, ensure that the evaluation team possesses) the education, abilities, skills, and experience appropriate to undertake the tasks proposed in the evaluation.

2 Evaluators should practice within the limits of their professional training and competence, and should decline to conduct evaluations that fall substantially outside those limits. When declining the commission or request that is not feasible or appropriate, evaluators should make clear any significant limitations on the evaluation that might result. Evaluators should make every effort to gain the competence directly or through the assistance of others who possess the required expertise.

3 Evaluators should continually seek to maintain and improve their competencies, in order to provide the highest level of performance in their evaluations. This continuing professional development

might include formal course work and workshops, self-study, evaluations of one's own practice, and working with other evaluators to learn from their skills and expertise.

Integrity/honesty

Evaluators ensure the honesty and integrity of the entire evaluation process.

1. Evaluators should negotiate honestly with clients and relevant stakeholders concerning the costs, tasks to be undertaken, limitations of methodology, scope of results likely to be obtained, and uses of data resulting from a specific evaluation. It is primarily the evaluator's responsibility to initiate discussion and clarification of these matters, not the clients'.
2. Evaluators should record all changes made in the originally negotiated project plans, and the reasons why the changes were made. If those changes significantly affect the scope and likely results of the evaluation, the evaluator should inform the client and other important stakeholders in a timely fashion (barring good reason to the contrary, before proceeding with further work) of the changes and their likely impact.
3. Evaluators should seek to determine, and where appropriate be explicit about, their own, their clients', and other stakeholders' interests concerning the conduct and outcomes of an evaluation (including financial, political, and career interests).
4. Evaluators should disclose any roles or relationships they have concerning whatever is being evaluated that might pose a significant conflict of interest with their role as an evaluator. Any such conflict should be mentioned in reports of the evaluation results.
5. Evaluators should not misrepresent their procedures, data, or findings. Within reasonable limits, they should attempt to prevent or correct any substantial misuses of their work by others.
6. If evaluators determine that certain procedures or activities seem likely to produce misleading evaluative information or conclusions, they have the responsibility to communicate their concerns, and the reasons for them, to the client (the one who funds or requests the evaluation). If discussions with the client do not resolve these concerns, so that a misleading evaluation is then implemented, the evaluator may legitimately decline to conduct the evaluation if that is feasible, and appropriate. If not, the evaluator should consult colleagues or relevant stakeholders about other proper ways to proceed (options might include, but are not limited to, discussion at a higher level, a dissenting cover letter or appendix, or refusal to sign the final document).

7 Barring compelling reasons to the contrary, evaluators should disclose all sources of financial support for an evaluation, and the source of the request for the evaluation.

Respect for people

Evaluators respect the security, dignity, and self-worth of the respondents, program participants, clients, and other stakeholders with whom they interact.

1 Where applicable, evaluators must abide by current professional ethics and standards regarding risks, harms, and burdens that might be engendered to those participating in the evaluation: regarding informed consent for participation in the evaluation; and regarding informing participants about the scope and limits of confidentiality. Examples of such standards include federal regulations about protection of human subjects, or the ethical principles of such associations as the American Anthropological Association, the American Educational Research Association, or the American Psychological Association. Although this principle is not intended to extend the applicability of such ethics and standards beyond their current scope, evaluators should abide by them where it is feasible and desirable to do so.

2 Because justified negative or critical conclusions from an evaluation must be explicitly stated, evaluations sometimes produce results that harm client or stakeholder interests. Under this circumstance, evaluators should seek to maximize the benefits and reduce any unnecessary harms that might occur, provided this will not compromise the integrity of the evaluation findings. Evaluators should carefully judge when the benefits from doing the evaluation or in performing certain evaluation procedures should be foregone because of the risks or harms. Where possible, these issues should be anticipated during the negotiation of the evaluation.

3 Knowing that evaluations often will negatively affect the interests of some stakeholders, evaluators should conduct the evaluation and communicate its results in a way that clearly respects the stakeholders' dignity and self-worth.

4 Where feasible, evaluators should attempt to foster the social equity of the evaluation, so that those who give to the evaluation can receive some benefits in return. For example, evaluators should seek to ensure that those who bear the burdens of contributing data and incurring any risks are doing so willingly, and that they have full knowledge of, and maximum feasible opportunity to obtain, any benefits that may be produced from

the evaluation. When it would not endanger the integrity of the evaluation, respondents or program participants should be informed if and how they can receive services to which they are otherwise entitled without participating in the evaluation.

5 Evaluators have the responsibility to identify and respect differences among participants, such as differences in their culture, religion, gender, abilities, age, sexual orientation and ethnicity, and to be mindful of potential implications of these differences when planning, conducting, analyzing, and reporting their evaluations.

Responsibilities for general and public welfare
Evaluators articulate and take into account the diversity of interests and values that may be related to the general and public welfare.

1 When planning and reporting evaluations, evaluators should consider including important perspectives and interests of the full range of stakeholders in the object being evaluated. Evaluators should carefully consider the justification when omitting important value perspectives or the views of important groups.

2 Evaluators should consider not only the immediate operations and outcomes of whatever is being evaluated, but also the broad assumptions, implications and potential side effects of it.

3 Freedom of information is essential in a democracy. Hence, barring a compelling reason to the contrary, evaluators should allow all relevant stakeholders to have access to evaluative information, and should actively disseminate that information to stakeholders if resources allow. If different evaluation results are communicated in forms that are tailored to the interests of different stakeholders, those communications should ensure that each stakeholder group is aware of the other communication. Communications that are tailored to a given stakeholder should always include all-important results that may bear on interests of that stakeholder. In all cases, evaluators should strive to present results as clearly and simply as accuracy allows so that clients and other stakeholders can easily understand the evaluation process and results.

4 Evaluators should maintain a balance between client needs and other needs. Evaluators necessarily have a special relationship with the client who funds or requests the evaluation. By virtue of that relationship, evaluators must strive to meet legitimate client needs whenever it is feasible and appropriate to do so. However, that relationship can also place evaluators in difficult dilemmas when client interests conflict with other interests, or when client

interests conflict with the obligation of evaluators for systematic inquiry, competence, integrity, and respect for people. In these cases, evaluators should explicitly identify and discuss the conflicts with the client and relevant stakeholders, resolve them when possible, determine whether continued work on the evaluation is advisable if the conflicts cannot be resolved, and make clear any significant limitations on the evaluation that might result if the conflict is not resolved.

5 Evaluators have obligations that encompass the public interest and good. These obligations are especially important when evaluators are supported by publicly generated funds; but clear threats to public good should never be ignored in any evaluation. Because the public interest and good are rarely the same as the interests of any particular group (including those of the client or funding agency), evaluators will usually have to go beyond an analysis of particular stakeholders' interests when considering the welfare of society as a whole.

The journal *New Directions for Program Evaluation* (Shadish et al 1995), devoted an edition to the discussion of the evolution and usage of the Guiding Principles and comparisons with the Program Evaluation Standards. A major contribution to this edition was an article by Sanders (1995), who compared the Program Evaluation Standards developed under his chairmanship with the Principles. He concluded that:

> I can safely say that there are no conflicts or inconsistencies between the two. Although there may be minor disagreements about where the AEA statements should be placed within the Joint Committee Standards, the overall advice is very consistent, with both documents strongly emphasizing accuracy of results, inclusion of stakeholders in the evaluation process, regard for the welfare of evaluation participants and a concern for service to stakeholders, the community and society. (Sanders 1995, p. 48)

Now that we have outlined the extensive work that has been done in this area, we would like to draw attention to a potential confusion of terminology. You may recall that in Chapter 1 we used the term 'standard' to refer to the required level of attainment on the scale of a variable as the basis for judging the worth of a program (or evaluand). It seems that to now use the term 'standard' to indicate the important parameters of acceptable practice is a little confusing. So, we will henceforth use the term 'codes of behavior' to refer collectively to the standards and to the guiding principles, and dimensions of acceptable professional practice.

APPLYING EVALUATION CODES OF BEHAVIOR

Of the major codes of behavior just described, the Program Evaluation Standards provide evaluators with more practical directions for use. One advantage is that, for each standard, there is a scale with the following anchor points:

- The standard was deemed applicable and to the extent feasible was taken into account.
- The standard was deemed applicable but could not be taken into account.
- The standard was not deemed applicable.
- Exception was taken to the standard.

The scale is used in a checklist to help evaluators determine whether the code of behavior for a given study is acceptable to clients. The availability of the documentation on the Standards is part of an impressive attempt by the developers to make them user-friendly. This is in recognition that the Standards are not only for the professional evaluator undertaking well-funded studies; they are also applicable to small-scale insider-for-insider studies.

As we indicated earlier in this chapter, the evaluator should be judicious in invoking the standards or principles. It is a mistake to think that they should be applied 'chapter and verse' in a slavish or unthinking way to an evaluation study.

An analysis of the use of the Standards shows that, very often, the standards of Accuracy and Feasibility can collide. For example, to get a very accurate estimate of population statistics, we may need a sample size so large that the survey becomes too expensive to undertake.

In this case, we may decide to use a smaller sample, knowing that the population estimate will vary considerably, or we may use key informants' estimates of the population size if they are likely to be sufficiently accurate for our purposes, or we may decide not to proceed until sufficient resources are available to undertake the large surveys required.

The Standards of Utility and Accuracy may also be at odds, particularly in terms of the trade-off between timeliness and comprehensiveness. It is sometimes important to provide a set of more tentative findings to the client in time to inform a key decision, rather than to assemble a more thorough analysis of the evidence which will only be available after the deadline.

An indicator of token or superficial evaluation is widespread non-compliance with the Standards. For example, studies that encourage changes in a program based only on client feedback data, using a small and unrepresentative sample of clients who volunteer to return evaluation surveys, violate standards belonging to both Accuracy and Utility.

As a minimum, we believe that all evaluators, whether they be professional evaluation consultants or graduate students working on a small-scale internal evaluation, should know what the Standards or principles contain and what they imply for a code of behavior.

APPLYING CODES OF BEHAVIOR TO REAL EVALUATIONS

It is a long step from getting people to understand a code of practice to having them internalize that code to the extent that it forms a basis for their action. Experience suggests that knowing about the Standards or principles is not enough: there is a need for them to be acted on. An obvious move is to encourage practitioners to use the codes in real evaluation studies. Beginning in the negotiation stage, it is up to the evaluator to take the initiative on their use.

This is why we have encouraged attention to codes of behavior in the evaluation planner outlined in Chapter 4 (see Figure 4.1). Negotiating should include determining which Standards should form part of the evaluation agreement and be included in the final evaluation plan. Where possible, the evaluator should look for any problems encompassed by the Standards that might arise in the data management and dissemination stages.

One of the problems in using the Standards has been to decide which of them should be used and when they would be most appropriately implemented during the course of an evaluation. We undertook an evaluation research study designed to simplify their use, as follows.

You will recall that we have described evaluation in terms of three elements:

- negotiation of an evaluation plan;
- development of an evaluation design; and
- dissemination of findings to identified audiences (see Chapter 1).

There is also a fourth element—the need for management of the evaluation project—which can be thought of as superordinate to the three elements just described. This has been discussed in Chapter 7 and relates to the smooth management and conduct of the study.

We asked a group of experienced evaluators and, separately, a group of postgraduate students, to allocate each Standard to one or more of the four evaluation elements just described. We deemed that, if 60 percent of the respondents assigned a given Standard to one of those elements, it 'belonged' to that element.

The results produced the following clusters:

- *Planning the evaluation.* The following Standards belonged to this element:
  U1: Stakeholder Identification
  F2: Political Viability
  P1: Service Orientation
  P2: Formal Agreements
  A1: Program Documentation
  A2: Context Analysis

- *Evaluation design.* The following Standards belonged to this element:
  F1: Practical Procedures
  P4: Human Interaction
  A6: Reliable Information
  A7: Systematic Information
  A8: Analysis of Quantitative Information
  A9: Analysis of Qualitative Information

- *Dissemination.* The following Standards belonged to this element:
  U4: Values Identification
  U5: Report Clarity
  U6: Report Timeliness and Dissemination
  P6: Disclosure of Findings
  A10: Justified Conclusions
  A11: Impartial Reporting

- *Managing the evaluation.* The following Standards belonged to this element:
  U7: Evaluation Impact
  F3: Cost Effectiveness
  P7: Conflict of Interest
  P8: Fiscal Responsibility
  A12: Metaevaluation

In all, 23 of the 30 Standards were allocated to these evaluation elements, leaving seven that belonged to more than one element on the criteria we set (Neale et al. 2003). Clustering the Standards in this way makes them easier to use, because it allocates them to evaluation stages that often follow sequentially, and may also be the responsibility of different members of an evaluation team. This applies in particular to the management element that is often the responsibility of the team leader.

USING PRINCIPLES IN TRAINING EVALUATORS

One way in which the use of codes of behavior can be encouraged is during the training of neophyte evaluators. A potential source of new evaluators is through formal graduate training in colleges and universities (Owen 1998). However, the general consensus is that most college courses in evaluation concentrate on methodology and do less than justice to many of the basic principles of evaluation practice, including an analysis of codes of behavior and their usage in real situations.

Worthen (1996), who has extensive experience in training evaluators in university settings, believes that codes of behavior for evaluation cannot be taught in isolation from more general concerns about ethics. He maintains that the inculcation of appropriate standards of practice must sensitize students to more general concerns about how we treat fellow human beings. Worthen believes that the formal training of evaluators should involve the modeling of appropriate behavior by university staff responsible for training. This implies that university staff must set high standards for the way they conduct themselves professionally and that they should be 'honest and upstanding'. Good training also involves teaching of standards and/or principles in an experiential format. This involves applying them, first of all, to simulated situations, and then to projects in the field. During this stage, students should be asked specifically to adhere to a code of behavior based on the standards or the guiding principles (Worthen 1996).

This implies a rigorous and extensive training program. There remains the problem of how those new to evaluation who do not have the benefit of extensive college training can apply codes of behavior to their work. There has been extensive discussion within the American Evaluation Society about ways in which the certification of evaluators might proceed. If there is a move towards certifying evaluations and evaluators, there will be a need to upgrade the quantity and quality of training for evaluators.

METAEVALUATION: USING THE STANDARDS OR PRINCIPLES TO REVIEW PRACTICE

Another way in which standards or principles can be used is as a framework for reviewing practice. This is known as metaevaluation, literally the evaluation of evaluations. The importance of metaevaluation is highlighted by the inclusion of Standard A12. Metaevaluations can be undertaken for different reasons. First, at a strategic time to check that a suitable code of behavior has been built in to a study from the beginning. This is the principle by which universities, colleges and other entities invoke the use of ethics committees.

Secondly, a metaevaluation is sometimes formally commissioned by an organization at the conclusion of a study to ensure that an evaluation it has supported has satisfied quality standards. The reviewer typically examines documents and interviews key stakeholders and the evaluation team. Thirdly, evaluators can undertake a 'self-metaevaluation' as part of reflective practice. In addition to the quality assurance outcome, the exercise provides an opportunity for the staff involved to 'get inside' the codes of behavior, and thus sharpen their understandings of this area as a basis for future evaluation work (Berends & Roberts 2003).

IMPACT ON THE FIELD

There is a dearth of empirical studies on the use of codes of behavior and factors affecting their use in the field. Two important studies are of note. The first asked a sample of experienced evaluators to rank the frequency of a set of violations to good practice, each one linked to one of the 30 standards in the Program Evaluation Standards. It was found that the respondents ranked Utility and Feasibility standards as more frequently violated than those of Accuracy and Propriety (Newman & Brown 1992).

A subsequent and more extensive study asked 700 members of the American Evaluation Association to report on their experiences with ethical problems in their work. An open-ended methodology was used to get respondents to describe:

- the ethical problems they had faced most frequently in their work; and
- the single most serious ethical problem they had ever encountered (Morris & Cohn 1993).

The 459 responses were subjected to content analyses, based on another set of principles, the Standards for Program Evaluation (SPE). The SPE consists of 66 principles, clustered under six headings:

- Formulation and Negotiation;
- Structure and Design;
- Data Collection and Preparation;
- Data Analysis and Interpretation;
- Communication and Disclosure;
- Use of Results.

It is worth noting that these principles, which are now largely superseded by those we have discussed above, correspond closely to the key steps in the evaluation planner (see Figure 4.1), which we introduced in Chapter 4.

Key findings of this study included the following:

- Almost 65 percent of respondents encountered ethical problems in their work.
- Ethical problems were more likely in external evaluations—that is, when the evaluator was an outsider.
- Ethical problems were more likely to be associated with process and outcome evaluations than with inquiry related to needs assessment or cost-benefit analysis.
- Evaluators who had a background in education were less likely to have encountered ethical problems than evaluators with backgrounds in other disciplines.

Most problems were located in the post-data management phase. They included:

- conflicts over the presentations of findings, such as pressure to alter a presentation, or being reluctant to fully outline findings due to their being at odds with the expectations of the client;
- disagreement over disclosure of findings, such as disputes concerning the ownership and dissemination of a final report; and
- misinterpretation or misuse of the final report, or the findings being suppressed or ignored by the client.

Morris and Cohn (1993) prepared a 'composite portrait' of an evaluator's nightmare, based on these findings:

> The client informs the evaluator at their initial meeting that it is extremely important to demonstrate that the program is having a significant beneficial effect on participants. Later, when the data indicate that the program's effects are not as positive as the client had hoped, the client exerts pressure on the evaluator to exaggerate the 'good' findings and downplay the 'bad' ones. At this point the client also questions the evaluator's right to discuss the findings with individuals outside of the organization, an issue the evaluator thought had been resolved during the contracting phase. Finally, after the final report has been submitted, the evaluator discovers that the document has been 'deep sixed'. The client has not shared it with other stakeholders within the agency, and does not appear to be using the study's results or recommendations in decision-making concerning the program (p. 639).

This has a familiar ring, reminding us of a study we undertook where the client was a federal government department. At the draft report stage, we received telephone calls from senior bureaucrats asking that the findings of an executive study be 'rearranged' by putting the more positive findings at the front, with the more negative ones relegated to the rear and downplayed. At about the same time, one of the evaluation team presented a report at a national education conference about some of the findings, which resulted in a threatening call from a senior bureaucrat to the director of the evaluation. Fortunately, after pressure from other stakeholders, some of the findings were distributed to the wide range of stakeholders; however, a major report with some criticisms of the roles of federal officers in liaising with their counterparts in the states was never released. The result of this and other studies suggest that ethical problems relate to the transmission of findings and their use, rather than to the negotiation and data management stages of an evaluation study.

CONCLUSION

Ernest House reviewed a series of evaluations undertaken by well-known evaluation agencies for the Federal Department of Education in Washington DC. He found that in none of these large-scale studies did evaluators or their clients ever broach ethical standards or principles. Our own experience of assisting public sector organizations is that codes of behavior do not get the exposure they warrant in the management of evaluation studies.

The application of codes of behavior still represents a major challenge for evaluation associations and their members. Professional associations have been proactive in encouraging the use of codes of behavior in evaluation practice. A notable manifestation of this has been the inclusion, over several years, of a section on Ethical Challenges in the *American Evaluation Journal*, edited by Michael Morris. The section poses an ethical case study problem and responses from well-known evaluators that outline how they would deal with the issue.

We have suggested several ways in which codes of behavior can be brought to the attention of new evaluators. We also believe that the more emphasis is placed on codes of behavior in the planning stage of evaluations, the more likely that stakeholders will become aware of them.

A further advantage of incorporating codes of behavior into the design of evaluations is that there will be fewer problems with ethical issues in the later stages of an evaluation. However, as others have pointed out, there is always the potential for conflict because of the basic difference in orientations of evaluators, concerned with the veracity of their evaluations, and managers, if the findings threaten the programs in which managers have a high stake (Kimmel 1988).

REFERENCES

Berends, L. and Roberts, B. (2003). Evaluation standards and their application to indigenous programs in Victoria, Australia. *Evaluation Journal of Australasia*, 3(2), 54–59.

Chelimsky, E. (1995). Comments of the guiding principles. *New Directions for Program Evaluation*, 66 (Summer), 53–59.

Fraser, D. (2001). Beyond ethics: Why we need evaluation standards. *Evaluation Journal of Australasia*, 1(1), 53–58.

Homan, R. (1991). *The Ethics of Social Research*. New York: Longman.

Kimmel, A. J. (1988). *Ethics and Values in Applied Social Research*. Newbury Park, CA: Sage.

Mirvis, P. H. and Seashore, S. E. (eds) (1982). *Creating Ethical Relationships in Organizational Research*. New York: Springer Verlag.

Morris, M. and Cohn, R. (1993). Program evaluation and ethical challenges: A national survey. *Evaluation Review*, 17, 621–42.

Neale, J., Owen, J. M. and Small, D. (2003). Encouraging the use of codes of behavior in evaluation practice. *Evaluation and Program Planning*, 26, 29–36.

Newman, D. L. and Brown, R. D. (1992). Violations of ethical standards: Frequency and seriousness of occurrence. *Evaluation Review*, 16, 219–34.

Owen, J. M. (1998). Towards an outcomes hierarchy for professional university programs. *Evaluation and Program Planning*, 21(3), 315–321.

Sanders, J. (1994). *The Program Evaluation Standards*. Thousand Oaks, CA: Sage.

Sanders, J. R. (1995). Standards and principles. *New Directions for Program Evaluation*, 66, 47–52.

Shadish, W. R., Newmann, D. L., Scheirer, M.A. and Wye, C. (eds) (1995). Developing the guiding principles. *New Directions for Program Evaluation*, 66, 3–18

Worthen, B. (1996). *Mechanisms for Making the Program Evaluation Standards Meaningful to Graduate Education*. Paper presented at the Annual Meeting of the American Evaluation Association, November 1996, Atlanta, GA.

Proactive Evaluation

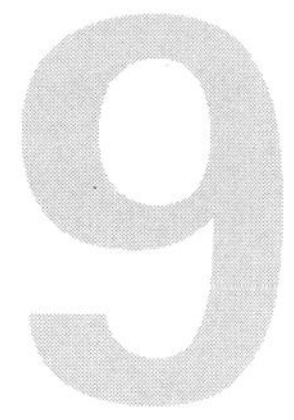

This chapter outlines the rationale and Approaches to evaluation designed to inform front-end decision-making about the structure and content of policies and programs. There are two major situations to which this Form of evaluation is logically applied. The first is in a 'nothing to something' situation where the aim of the evaluation is to provide findings to aid decision-making about a new program, one being developed from scratch. In the second, a program exists but there is a need for a major review, with the likelihood that this existing program will be altered radically or even replaced by a new and more appropriate one.

Because, in both instances, these evaluations provide information in order to assist decisions about a future or projected program, evaluations of this nature are described as Proactive evaluations.

Proactive evaluation is concerned with:

- the extent of the need among a defined population for a program in a given area of provision;
- synthesizing what is known in the existing research and related literature about an identified issue or problem; and
- critically reviewing ways in which an identified issue or problem has been solved through programs mounted in other locations.

The essential features of Proactive evaluation are summarized in Table 9.1.

Table 9.1 shows that the *orientation*, or purpose of evaluation, of a Proactive evaluation is to provide findings to aid the synthesis of programs. Given that the *state* of these programs is that either no program exists or that radical changes are needed to an existing one, the timing of the evaluation can be conceived of as occurring 'before development'. The *focus* from which evidence is drawn is the

Table 9.1 Summary of Proactive evaluation

Dimension	Properties
Orientation	Synthesis
Typical issues	• Is there a need for the program? • What do we know about this problem that the program will address? • What is recognized as best practice in this area? • Have there been other attempts to find solutions to this problem? • What does the relevant research or conventional wisdom tell us about this problem? • What could we find out from external sources to rejuvenate an existing policy or program?
State of program	None
Major focus	Program context
Timing (vis-à-vis program delivery)	Before
Key Approaches	• Needs assessment • Research synthesis • Review of best practice (establishment of benchmarks)
Assembly of evidence	Questionnaire, review of documents and data bases, site visits and other interactive methods. Focus groups, nominal groups and delphi technique useful for needs assessments.

context or milieu within which the program will or may be developed, or like contexts in other locations.

Employing Approaches within this Form assumes that policy and program development should be informed by the best and most appropriate evidence about the problem to be addressed. For example, an analysis of needs, combined with information on available resources, is fundamental to making decisions about the provision of services. Such knowledge enables planners at the policy, Program and program levels to:

- determine priorities in geographic areas, among client groups and across areas of support;
- train and allocate staff appropriately;
- locate services and facilities to achieve maximum effect;
- substantiate the allocation of resources.

The evaluator's task is to harness and provide knowledge for those who will be involved in program planning. The logic for Proactive evaluation seems to be beyond challenge. In practice, however, examples of its application to real life are hard to locate. This suggests that decisions related to planning interventions have traditionally been based on the intuition of program staff, long-used practices, personal preferences, or have been unduly influenced by political pressures. The use of evaluation to aid decision-making before programs are developed is a call for a more analytical and rational approach to the allocation of precious resources such as those applied to social and educational interventions.

KEY APPROACHES TO PROACTIVE EVALUATION

Three major Approaches to Proactive evaluation (see Table 9.1) are:

- needs assessment;
- research synthesis (evidence-based practice); and
- review of exemplary practice (and the establishment of benchmarks).

  Each of these Approaches will now be considered in turn.

Needs assessment

Needs assessment is a well-established Approach. An extensive conceptual literature has emerged, and the American Evaluation Association has a strong Topical Interest Group on needs assessment, an indication that this Approach is acknowledged as an important subset of evaluation practice. A needs assessment is defined as:

> A systematic set of procedures undertaken for the purpose of setting priorities and making decisions about program or organizational improvements and allocation of resources. The priorities are based on identified needs (Witkin & Altschuld 1995).

To undertake a needs assessment, one must come to grips with the notion of a *need*. This is not an easy notion to deal with, as there are many views on what we actually mean by a need (Scriven 1991). Using 'need' as a noun provides a basis for defining what is meant by needs assessment. Need is the difference between the desired and the present situation or condition. Need is thus a discrepancy. This contrasts with the use of the term 'need' in everyday parlance as a verb. Using 'need' as a verb focuses on solutions—for example, a community might say:

'We need a new health center in the neighborhood'. We are now talking about the program to fix the need, rather than the investigation that should precede it. According to Witkin and Altschuld (1995), these two meanings are often confounded, and it is essential that the notion of need as a discrepancy remains uppermost in the minds of those commissioning or undertaking needs assessments.

Spelling out the essential features of a need leads us to be concerned with five elements, as follows:

- the desired or ideal condition or state of affairs, or what ought to be;
- the present or actual condition or state of affairs;
- discrepancies between desired and actual conditions;
- reasons for the discrepancies; and
- deciding which needs should be given priority for action through a treatment or program.

According to Roth (1990), need can be generally defined as follows:

$$N = D - A$$

where N is the need or discrepancy, D is the desired state and A is the actual state. Roth has shown that need is not a unitary concept. There are different meanings as indicated in Table 9.2.

Table 9.2 Different meanings of 'need'

N		D		A
Goal discrepancy	=	ideal state	–	actual state
Social discrepancy	=	normative state	–	actual state
Essential discrepancy	=	minimal state of acceptability	–	actual state
Want discrepancy	=	desired state	–	actual state

For each of these situations, the desired state differs and thus, in a given context, the discrepancy will be different, both in nature and amount. For example, the gap between the minimal and actual state would be smaller than that between ideal and actual. Note that in the fourth of these definitions, there is a shift from needs to wants. It is important to distinguish a need from a want. An example may clarify this.

Example 9.1 Undertaking a needs assessment in a school of nursing

The example is organized around the five stages outlined above:

1 the desired or ideal state of affairs;
2 the present or actual state of affairs;
3 discrepancies between 1 and 2;
4 reasons for the needs or discrepancies; and
5 which need should be given priority for action through a treatment or program.

Imagine that a review is being undertaken of teaching methods in a school of nursing which has a reputation for being conservative. An agenda for the evaluation, sponsored by the managing committee of the school, is to make the school more responsive to recent developments in teaching and learning.

One possibility is to carry out a wants discrepancy.

1 An evaluator is asked to review the actual methods used. This is done through observation of classes and interviews with teachers.
2 At the same time, the evaluator surveys nurse education teachers working in the school about teaching methods they would prefer to use.
3 The evaluator determines differences between the actual and desired state. The analysis shows that there is little difference between methods used and preferences expressed.
4 The evaluator notes the size and the nature of the (wants) discrepancy. Some comments about the reasons or causes for the discrepancy are given on the basis of the knowledge of the context of the evaluation.
5 The evaluator presents his or her conclusions about the size and nature of the discrepancy to the management committee. The committee notes the findings, which imply minor policy and practice changes.

A second possibility is to carry out a social discrepancy.

1 The evaluator also reviews the latest guidelines on effective nursing teaching which appear in educational documents and visits other like schools to determine methods commonly in use.
2 This stage is identical to that undertaken in the wants assessment.

3 On the basis of this information the evaluator prepares a statement of an 'ideal' state for teaching in the school, a direction to work towards through staff development. This is the social discrepancy.
4 The evaluator notes the size and the nature of the (needs) discrepancy. Some comments about the reasons or causes for the discrepancy are given on the basis of the knowledge of the context of the evaluation.
5 The evaluator presents his or her conclusions about the size and nature of the discrepancy to the management committee. The committee notes the findings, which imply major policy and practice changes. Among them is the need for new directions in teaching practice and a program of professional development for teaching staff.

Comparing the two assessments

If both assessments were carried out, the evaluator could note that the two discrepancies are very different both in size and nature. Some comments about the reasons or causes for each discrepancy could be given on the basis of the knowledge of the context of the evaluation. Decisions about action by the committee would depend on their collective opinions about which of the two assessments is more valid in terms of the aims or mission of the school.

The existence of these two types of needs can be explained by the context within which the evaluations are conducted. Determination of what ought to be is the basis for each discrepancy. What ought to be depends on the frame of reference for the evaluation. Needs assessments, like other evaluations, are political activities. Needs or wants are conditional. In the social discrepancy example above, the need for staff development is conditional on the assumption that more up-to-date teaching methods are required. In this case, establishment of the need comes down to the need for students in the nurse education programs to learn more effectively.

Needs assessment in practice has three major stages: planning, data management and utilization. This is consistent with our description of evaluation introduced in Chapter 1. The planning stage culminates in a management plan, which includes the purposes of the study, an outline of the methods to be adopted, and the potential uses of the findings. Data management includes locating existing sources of information—often an important source of data for needs assessments—and the collection of new evidence. This must include evidence about both the actual and desired conditions. In the utilization stage, needs are prioritized if competing needs have been found. In some cases, action plans to ameliorate the needs are developed. In these cases, there is a strong link between the evaluative and development aspects of program provision. This involves evaluators working closely with clients and adopting an insider-for-insider perspective on the evaluation (see Chapter 7).

It is essential that all three stages are included for a study to be classed as a needs assessment. Reviews of the field have shown that studies often fall short of one or more of these criteria. These studies showed that major shortcomings included:

- confusing solutions with needs;
- not attending to the establishment of the desired state or condition;
- relying on one method of data collection, usually a questionnaire;
- equating the administration of a questionnaire with the needs assessment;
- failing to attend to the establishment of needs;
- neglecting to assist clients with setting priorities for action (Witkin & Altschuld 1995).

Research synthesis (evidence-based practice)

A second Approach within the Proactive evaluation Form is research synthesis, or *evidence-based practice* (EBP). The case for EBP rests on the same assumptions as the other Approaches in this chapter.

Simply put, the rationale for EBP is: that which has been previously discovered through systematic inquiry should be applied to the development and implementation of a new intervention. EBP can be seen as a 'scientific' response to program planning, with a status above other influences such as the craft knowledge of practitioners, and local knowledge about the context in which the program is to be introduced.

At the level of principle, this rationale is persuasive. Governments have supported the emergence of EBP as a means by which the funds they expend on pure and applied research can provide more tangible benefits to society. The use of EBP also suits the neo-liberal agenda of more control over public policy. Potentially, EBP supports the case for more central authority over decision-making, with the unfortunate corollary of discouraging experimentation and diversity among program providers.

Synthesizing evidence to inform professional practice emerged within the medical fraternity, where the concept of *evidence-based medicine* (EBM) has become influential. Originally, individual medical practitioners were encouraged to search, summarize and use research literature. Now, however, responsibilities for searching and summarizing research have passed to specialized central agencies which disseminate findings to practitioners. There are many Internet sites which provide support for EBM. Databases such as EBM Online and bodies such as the Center for Disease Control and Prevention are working to improve the implementation of EBM.

The trends observable among the medical professions now permeate other public policy areas such as health, welfare and education. For example, the British-based Centre for Evidence-Based Policy and Practice has been extensively supported in terms of its roles as a synthesizer of research, and research on utilization of EBM (http://www.evidencenetwork.org/). The expansion of evidence-based practice from medicine to other areas of public provision has led to an increased interest among social scientists and the application of previous accumulated research into knowledge utilization dating back for at least two decades (Heller 1986).

EBP knowledge production

The 'rational' EBP model assumes a *research-into-practice* approach to change, through which the synthesis of findings undertaken by 'remotely located' researchers is transmitted and applied to the world of practitioners.

The intention of early proponents of EBP was to encourage the use of rigorously produced scientific knowledge into policy decision-making. Influenced by the medical perspective, a hierarchy of methods of knowledge production has emerged. At the top is the controlled random experiment, followed by other 'lesser' methods in order—quasi-experiments, cohort studies, case studies, consensus, and experience and opinion. The focus of these studies is on outcomes for participants and the conditions that promote them; they are known as 'process–outcome studies'.

For a policy-maker or practitioner wishing to apply this Approach to decision-making about a proposed program, it is necessary to gain access to the findings of a previously completed synthesis, or commission someone to perform a tailored synthesis of relevant studies. Two methods of synthesis appear in the literature:

- numerical meta-analysis; and
- narrative reviews (Pawson 2002).

Both rely on the identification of a 'family of programs' that bear similarity to the one being proposed by the policy-maker.

Meta-analysis relies heavily on findings from studies employing experimental or quasi-experimental designs. The evaluator identifies sub-types of the program, on the basis of the same or similar modes of delivery. Outcomes of programs within each sub-type are aggregated before comparisons across sub-types are made using the statistical concept of 'effect size'. The strategy then ranks the effects of these programs, thus providing the policy-maker with information to be used in deciding on the way the new program will be developed and implemented.

The *narrative review*, or *descriptive-analytical method*, is based on the development and use of a template to analyze a family of programs. It relies on the use of qualitative interpretation of key aspects, including details of implementation attributes, and thus provides detailed analysis of how programs work. While the production of matrices containing these aspects can be thought of as the end point of the synthesis, Pawson (2002) exhorts the analysts to go the extra mile and undertake interpretations of the matrix entries, and provides guidelines on how to do so (pp. 176–179).

While there are some theorists who continue to support the exclusive adoption of the random experiment as the only basis for EBP, most social program evaluators recognize that this is often impractical. For example, Rog (2003) reported an EBP study that was designed to provide guidance on supported housing policy. In addition to quasi-experimental studies, she interrogated studies that used other methods, such as multi-site case studies. Access to these findings involved a review of published and unpublished studies, which highlights the issue of gaining access to relevant studies. Rog believes that her work showed the value of synthesis, even in areas where the existing research was 'not perfect'. She also noted that, even where the data sets were complete, there were gaps in the knowledge required by the policy-maker. While the steps in her analyses are not available, it is likely that a variation in narrative review was used, in that she was able to report data sets on operational (implementation) issues in addition to outcomes.

The discussion above may help us understand why EBP has had less impact on social and educational program decisions than one might expect. Issues include:

- the ability to identify clearly the area of policy development envisaged;
- the possibility that no similar programs have been previously implemented;
- the possibility that, even if similar programs have been previously implemented, they have not been subject to rigorous evaluation, and hence there is insufficient evidence from which to synthesize findings.

Taken together, these issues point to a fundamental assumption about the use of EBP, which is that the phenomenon or problem being addressed has been subject to similar program interventions previously. This is patently not always the case, evidenced by the extensive literature on innovation development and diffusion. Social program innovations are, by definition, novel attempts to solve identified problems, innovative practice is often ahead of policy and related research agendas.

If we assume that a synthesis of relevant evidence does exist, we need to locate it among the wide variety of EBP providers now found in social science (including evaluator) communities. If this synthesis does not exist, the commissioner of the synthesis evaluation needs to commission a tailored study and deal with:

- clarifying the nature and boundaries of the study; and
- employing an evaluation team which can locate relevant studies and has the ability to analyze them in ways consistent with the methods described above.

While the emphasis in EBP has been on process–outcome studies—in other words, on what works—many social scientists see this as limiting the range of knowledge that can be synthesized. Other topics relevant to effective policy and program provision that research synthesis could focus on include:

- 'know-about' problems—for example, about current directions in an area of social policy;
- 'know-how' to implement interventions;
- 'know-whom' to involve, in order to implement successful interventions;
- 'know-why' programs are required.

Techniques for performing syntheses of these kinds have been undertaken but codification of relevant methods is still required (Ekblom 2001).

As we have indicated, traditional EBP and research synthesis more generally are predicated on a *research-into-practice* model. This can be contrasted with a *research-in-practice* model, in which the generation of evidence and professional practice are more closely linked. A research-in-practice model encourages practitioners to undertake meaningful research on their own practice, related to their own agendas, and is consistent with an Interactive Form of evaluation discussed in depth in Chapter 11.

However, there is no doubt that policy-making on many fronts would benefit from research syntheses which, while acknowledging their limitations, can provide directions for action. A key issue for those who support the use of Proactive evaluation is for managers and others associated with policy-making to see the potential value of spending resources on proactive studies that tap the findings of previous relevant research.

Given that this Approach is about research synthesis, we have focused here on the ways in which research-into-practice could benefit policy development. While EBP supporters were initially concerned about the quality of the knowledge *produced* by these processes, there has been an expansion of concern about factors such as *dissemination* and *use* of the products of research, in effect on the impact of EBP on organizational and policy/program decision-making. Proponents of EBP now understand that they have to devise more effective strategies for disseminating research and its integration into policy-making processes.

> The traditional research-into-practice model is uni-dimensional, plotting the course of research from creation through dissemination to utilization, and emphasizing linearity and logic. This is viewed as a rational but far from easy process, and the literature identifies many factors that may intercede along the way to hinder research utilization . . . More recently, knowledge use has been reconceptualized as a learning process, in which new knowledge is shaped by the learner's pre-existing knowledge and experience . . . Knowledge use is a complex change process in which 'getting the research out there' is only the first step . . . This involves paying attention not just to new knowledge (from research) but also to understanding how practitioner problems are conceptualized in relation to existing practitioner knowledge (Nutley et al. 2003).

This observation reminds us that the application of findings from a research synthesis will not be the sole input into policy or program decision-making. It should be noted that the notion of evidence-based medicine (EBM) is now assumed to involve the combined use of clinical research *and* clinical experience (craft knowledge) to make considered decisions about the best course of action for the treatment of patients. This combination should also apply to effective social program planning, to acknowledge the contribution of understandings beyond those gained from the research synthesis. In this respect, research on EBP and that on evaluation use shows considerable overlap, which strengthens a case for EBP being regarded as an Approach to evaluation, and which, due to its timing, must be included within the Proactive Form.

Review of best practice (establishment of benchmarks)

There is no doubt that benchmarking was one of the buzzwords or vogue terms in management in the 1990s (Bendell et al. 1993). Basically, benchmarking is the search for best practices that can be applied with a view to achieving improved performance. Benchmarking is a systematic and continuous process of measuring and comparing an organization's business processes against those of leaders anywhere in the world, to gain information which will help drive continuous improvement (Sharp 1994).

Establishment of benchmarks in industry is consistent with the idea of 'a continuous systematic process of evaluating companies that are recognized as industry leaders, to determine business and work processes that represent best practices and establish rational performance goals' (Cross & Iqbal 1994). Benchmarking involves systematic processes which involve searching for, introducing and implementing best practice. The search may focus on any of the major types of evaluands: organizations, policies, programs, services or products (Evans 1994).

Because of the focus of this book, we concentrate on one particular type of benchmarking that relies on the use of evidence collected directly from organizationally specific comparisons (Sharp 1994) or from secondary sources, such as databases (MacNeil et al. 1994). Cases of 'best practice' are located and identified, and the principles documented as an input to developing policies or programs based on the findings. This may involve comparisons with competitors. The documentation is the basis for assisting an organization to create, implement and monitor programs based on the principles identified in the best practice cases.

A key is to locate practitioners who have shown that their practice has a superior edge in the provision of services or products in a given area. If possible, a range of case examples should be used to assemble evidence. Inductive methods of analysis are used to draw out the underlying assumptions and principles of action across the cases.

This Approach is based on an assumption that best or innovatory practice in the workplace should be disseminated and used more widely (Spendolini 1992). Procedures must be employed to capture and transfer this knowledge to other users. The evaluator's role can be thought of as synthesizing evidence from cases located at the hub of a wheel. Assembling the findings is akin to the evidence traveling inwards on spokes to the hub. Policies and programs are synthesized at the hub and are disseminated to other practitioners via other spokes of the wheel.

Initially popular in business, benchmarking has more recently been applied to the provision of government services. While a range of interpretations exists, benchmarking by an organization generally includes the following stages:

1 identification of the area of operation to be benchmarked;
2 identification of best practice in selected organizations or sections of organizations;
3 collection and analysis to determine the common characteristics of this practice;
4 development of best practice indicators and levels to be achieved on these indicators;
5 communication of best practice indicators internally and gaining of acceptance;
6 development and implementation of plans to achieve these levels;
7 progress monitoring; and
8 full integration of practice into the functioning of the organization.

The organization could move through these stages again at a later time, with a focus on a different area of operation.

For the purposes of this discussion, we divide the benchmarking process into two phases. The first relates to stages 1–4, the second to stages 4–8. We regard stages 1–4 as the establishment of benchmarks, while stages 5–8 represent the application of benchmarks to the operations of an organization. In this Approach we are concerned only with the *establishment* of benchmarks, as this is consistent with an 'evaluation for development' perspective of the Proactive Form. The *application* of benchmarks falls within the study of Monitoring evaluation Form (see Chapter 12).

Simply described, the establishment of benchmarks attempts to answer the following questions:

- Who is doing best?
- How do they do it?
- How well are we doing relative to the best?
- How good do we want to be, relative to the best?

In more formal terms, benchmarking establishment involves an organization in:

- the targeted identification of best practice, and a consideration of whether this practice applies to the organization;
- a thorough, sustained program of external analysis and investigation; and
- the ability to reduce the findings of best practice to indicators that are meaningful as a management tool within the organization.

PROACTIVE EVALUATION: TRENDS AND CASE STUDIES

Use of creative data management

Assembling findings by the collection and analysis of evidence is an integral part of all evaluation studies. While the underlying principles of assembling evidence are the same across Forms, certain methods are more likely to be useful for a given Form. Table 9.1 presents a summary of useful ways in which evidence can be assembled for studies that fit within the Proactive Form. As we have indicated earlier, more than one type of data collection is usually required.

Example 9.2 Workplace communication

A government department was preparing to develop a workplace basic education project, in which classes in reading, writing and oral communication could be provided during work time for employees. An important objective was to develop a program that would be responsive to the changing needs of industry, while at the same time acknowledging the need for a basic education for working people. It was important to locate workplaces where the need for such a program was greatest, and to use the most effective teaching strategies.

A needs assessment was the means of assembling information by which a responsive program could be developed. To determine the 'desired state', it was decided that a better knowledge of communication requirements in the workplace was necessary. A group of service providers agreed to support an evaluation team to identify and investigate workplace communication. The result was an in-depth review of the communication needs of workers on the job. Later, the 'existing state' of the workers' communication skills was established by administering a series of tests. This allowed an analysis of the gaps in the existing communication skills of the workers. The findings were used to plan a program that was designed to reduce the gap between the actual and desired situations.

In a more extensive study in the area of community-oriented needs assessment, Neuber (1980) used the following sources:

- information from public records to create demographic statistical profiles. The profiles included birth and death rates, and statistics on employment, crime and mental health;

- key informants, defined as people having direct contact with individuals having problems with their lifestyles. Random samples were drawn from several relevant populations, including doctors, school counsellors and social agencies;
- consumers, for in community-orientated needs assessment, consumers must be consulted. Data were collected by individually interviewing a random sample of the adult population in the geographical area served by the projected program or service.

By focusing on similar issues using different methodologies and data sources, Neuber was more certain of his conclusions than if the information had been obtained from one source only.

Generally, there is a need for investigatory and inductive methodologies within the Proactive Form through the use of creative and unique ways of assembling evidence that are not usually adopted in other Forms. These methods are designed to gauge opinions of key players, gain consensus about the desired state for a prospective program, or plot a direction for action. These include:

- *Delphi technique*. This term is applied to methodology in which respondents work independently to pool their written ideas about a relevant issue. Each person is then given a copy of the collected ideas, appropriately developed into a set of scaled items, and asked to assess their relative importance. There is often more than one round of assessment, with the view of obtaining consensus (Dixon & Harding 1990).

Example 9.3 Needs of staff employed in the welding industry

The Edison Welding Institute (EWI) is an umbrella organization representing the interests of member companies and the welding industry at large in the United States. EWI employed an evaluation team to undertake a Delphi study of immediate and future educational needs of welding staff.

Preliminary discussions were held with stakeholders to determine the major purposes of the study and the methodology to be used, including sampling.

The purposes of the study were to:

- identify critical education and training needs that could be addressed by the company within six to twelve months (immediate needs) and during the next three years (future needs);

- rank-order each set of needs according to priorities of EWI member organizations;
- obtain respondents' comments about these needs; and
- provide this information for use in planning EWI programs.

Regarding sampling, questionnaires were sent to official representatives of EWI member organizations across the United States. In addition, the project identified companies which might fall under the umbrella of the EWI in the future and sought the information from them.

Regarding methodology, the Delphi technique was reviewed and approved by the stakeholders of the project. It was decided to concentrate on industry-wide, rather than company-specific, problems as the basis for structuring the data collection.

Official representatives of EWI member organizations were initially contacted by telephone, as a means of establishing and maintaining a high degree of cooperation and commitment from the respondents. This strategy was based on research which showed that questionnaires work best when a bond is formed between respondents and evaluators. Approximately 300 telephone calls were made to 108 companies.

Representatives of the Institute across the country participated in the two Delphi rounds. In the first, an open-ended questionnaire encouraged respondents to offer ideas about immediate and future training needs. About 30 immediate problems and 40 future needs were synthesized from this procedure. A feature of the analysis was the use of technical knowledge of EWI staff to make sense of the problems and needs suggested by the respondents.

Based on these responses, a second questionnaire was developed. Respondents were asked to read 30 needs statements related to immediate problems, and to identify the seven most important. Space was also provided for respondents to comment on the items and to suggest additional items. An identical procedure was used for the 40 future needs statements. The analysis consisted of simple tabulations of rankings of these responses.

The study reported the following:

- Twenty-nine immediate problems and 40 future needs were synthesized from the results of the first questionnaire.
- High priority immediate and future education and training needs were identified by ranking 62 responses to the second questionnaire. Few comments or additional educational and training problems were submitted.

The study thus provided EWI with base data for establishing both immediate and future education and training needs. In addition, the evaluators indicated that needs of employers were likely to change and that the Institute should consider routinely assessing the needs of its members. (Thomas & Altschuld 1985)

- *Search conference.* A search conference is an event designed to provide direction to a projected program or policy. Program staff and administration are involved in a search for appropriate solutions, given their knowledge of the context in which the program is to be developed and delivered. To be effective, such a conference must be carefully planned and custom designed. A search conference is based on an assumption that people want to create their own futures, and that they will act creatively and purposefully to achieve this end. In a search conference, participants will be engaged in issues such as: Where have we come from? Where do we want to go? What are the barriers and drivers to achieving desirable programs and activities? Participants are engaged in these questions as they relate to contextual issues and the system or organization in which they work (Emery 1990).
- *Nominal group forum.* The nominal group Approach was developed to assist people to deal with problems, set priorities and review possibilities. The four essential stages of nominal group method are:

  1. generation of ideas;
  2. recording of each idea;
  3. discussion of the ideas; and
  4. voting on the ideas.

- *Concept mapping.* Concept mapping is a technique used by groups to develop an understanding of a context in order to guide program planning. The term 'structured conceptualization' is used to define processes that involve a sequence of operationally defined steps leading to a conceptual representation of the context. There are six steps in concept mapping. These are:

  1. preparation, which includes the selection of participants and the development of a focus to the exercise;
  2. the generation of statements about the focus;
  3. structuring these statements;
  4. using statistical techniques such as multi-dimension scaling and cluster analysis to represent these statements as cluster maps;
  5. interpretation of the maps; and
  6. utilization of findings and organizational learning (Sutherland & Katz 2005).

- *Focus group*. The focus group is a technique designed to collect information about an issue from a small group of selected people through group discussion. Compared with Delphi, where consensus is the desired outcome, the aim of focus groups is to get a range of views on an issue. The focus group has its origins in the work of Merton et al. (1956). In this seminal work, *The Focused Interview*, Merton found that valid and useful information could be collected from a small group of people through the creation of a relaxed and permissive environment. A key aspect of focus groups is the use of an expert moderator. The Approach used in groups is to move from broader to more specific and substantive issues through the discussion. As with all data management techniques, the quality of data collection and analysis is crucial to the process. The technique has assumed wide popularity, encouraging innovative uses—for example, through use of the telephone as the medium for the assembly of evidence (Hurworth 2004).

Proactive evaluation as an agent of change

As indicated earlier, Proactive evaluation can support radical changes to an existing policy that is seen to be out of date or not serving the needs of those for whom it was intended. The following is an example of this scenario in which a research review was the evaluation Approach used.

Example 9.4 Is the music curriculum in dire straits?

Policy-makers in a state department of education and the arts were concerned about the content and practice in the teaching of music in government schools. While most schools offered music programs, some officials believed that the curriculum was unresponsive to the needs of the large majority of students. An evaluation study was commissioned to investigate the accuracy of these perceptions and to provide guidelines for a revision of music curriculum policy. An important aspect of the evaluation was a major review of recent research on essential elements of school music programs designed to respond to the interests and needs of young people. The review involved a computer-based literature search of worldwide publications in the area, an analysis of recent national documentation, and interviews with music curriculum personnel in the department and in selected schools. An extensive review was written, based on the material collected (Stringer & Owen 1986).

The next example is also one where the study was designed to encourage change to the status quo. In this case, the Approach used was a best practice review, rather than a research synthesis. The use of this Approach requires the evaluator to identify examples of best practice from which to collect evidence. This involves the selection of sites and is basically a question of sampling. The evaluator may have to develop criteria or the advice of experts when selecting sites, as was the case here.

Example 9.5 Youth culture and the arts

This study, funded through a national arts project, was designed to document ways in which teachers of the arts incorporated the interests of youth into the curriculum of the senior secondary school. Evidence included eight case studies of exemplary practice in schools in four states. A set of criteria was assembled and arts consultants in these states were asked to identify teachers whose practice was consistent with these criteria. The sites were visited throughout the school year to discover the essential characteristics of the programs and to identify factors which led to their development. The data were used in a cross-site analysis to discover common features of the innovative programs. This was the subject of a major report that was distributed to policy-makers and schools.

Impetus of benchmarking

Supporting best practice by both the private and public sectors has become a major theme in most Western democracies over the past decade. This has been fueled by global competition and the need for these democracies to be competitive and maintain standards of living for their citizens.

Example 9.6 The Australian Best Practice Program

Announced by the Federal Government in March 1991, the program's objectives were to:

- stimulate Australian enterprises to adopt international best practice;

- identify effective methods and approaches for the implementation of best practice in Australian enterprises; and
- promote a wider understanding of best practice and the benefits of its adoption by Australian enterprises.

The program had two components:

- *funding best practice projects within companies* which were used as role models for industry. Funding included a demonstration element which required companies to share their experiences with others in the business community. This included hosting visits, speaking at seminars, and preparing case studies.
- *dissemination of experiences*, including a comprehensive program of conferences, seminars and site visits across the country.

Benchmarking has also influenced the public sector. There are promising signs of the creative development and use of benchmarks within local government. In a small-scale study, it was found that city councils responded to a national benchmarking project by comparing the way they undertook the provision of services with other councils known to be leaders in the area. One council concentrated on services such as parks and gardens maintenance, valuations and drainage. The other concentrated on its election processes, community consultation and community grants.

There are indications that the evaluative aspect of benchmarking initiatives has been hampered by a lack of internal evaluative skills in both the private and public sectors. This will have to be ameliorated if the full effect of transferability of quality practice implied in the benchmarking movement is to be transferred across systems embracing its ideals.

CONCLUSION

This chapter discusses the Proactive Form of evaluation. Such evaluations are sometimes known as 'up-front', in that they are undertaken before policies and programs are planned and implemented. The role of the evaluator is to marshal evidence and provide findings which will assist in decision-making about whether a program should be mounted and, if so, the content and strategies to adopt in a given social intervention.

As with all evaluations, it is important that Proactive evaluation be responsive to the concerns of the client, which in this case is likely to be the potential program developer. Three major Approaches and some methodological techniques have been outlined. The choice and combination of Approaches and methodologies must be made with knowledge of an individual situation. This is up to the evaluator, in consultation with the client, to decide. In Proactive evaluation, novel data management techniques can be employed. There is clearly a need for expertise in 'up-front' evaluation Approaches and opportunities currently exist for evaluators to specialize in this Form of evaluation.

REFERENCES

Bendell, T., Boulter, L. and Kelly, J. (1993). *Benchmarking for Competitive Advantage*. London: Pitman Publishing.

Cross, R. and Iqbal, A. (1994). The Rank Xerox experiment: Benchmarking ten years on. In A. Rolstadas (ed.), *Benchmarking: Theory and Practice*. London: Chapman & Hall, 3–10.

Dixon, J. and Harding, G. (1990). DELPHI forecasting methodology. In *Proceedings of the National Conference of the Australasian Evaluation Society*, 1. Sydney, 255–258.

Ekblom, P. (2001). From source to the mainstream is uphill. *Cited in* S. Nutley, I. Walter and H. T. O. Davies, (2003), From knowing to doing. *Evaluation*, 9(2), 128.

Emery, M. (1990). The search conference as evaluation planning. In *Proceedings of the National Evaluation Conference of the Australasian Evaluation Society*. 1. Sydney, 259–262.

Evans, A. (1994). *Benchmarking*. Melbourne: Information Australia.

Heller, F. (1986). Introduction and Overview. In F. Heller (ed.), *The Use and Abuse of Social Science*. London: Sage, 4–6.

Hurworth, R. E. (2004). Telephone Focus Groups. *Social Research Update, Sociology at Surrey, University of Surrey*, 1–4.

MacNeil, J., Testi, J., Cupples, J. and Rimmer, M. (1994). *Benchmarking Australia*. Melbourne: Longman.

Merton, R. K., Fiske, M. and Kendall, P. L. (1956). *The Focused Interview*. Glencoe, MA: The Free Press.

Neuber, K. A. (1980). *Needs Assessment: A Model for Community Planning*. Beverly Hills, CA: Sage.

Nutley, S., Walter, I. and Davies, H. T. O. (2003). From knowing to doing. *Evaluation*, 9(2), 125–148.

Pawson, R. (2002). Evidence-based policy: In search of a method. *Evaluation*, 8(2), 157–181.

Rog, D. J. (2003). *Developing an Evidence Base that Guides Practice: When is the Level of Evidence Good Enough?* Paper presented at the annual meeting of the American Evaluation Association, Reno, NV.

Roth, J. (1990). Needs and the needs assessment process. *Evaluation Practice*, 11(2), 39–44.

Scriven, M. (1991). *Evaluation Thesaurus*, 4th ed. Newbury Park, CA: Sage.

Sharp, C. A. (1994). Industry best-practice benchmarking in the evaluation context. *Evaluation News and Comment*, 3(1), 27–33.

Spendolini, M. J. (1992). *The Benchmarking Book*. New York: AMACOM.

Stringer, W. and Owen, J. M. (1986). *Is the Music Curriculum in Dire Straits?* Melbourne: Centre for Program Evaluation, Melbourne College of Advanced Education.

Sutherland, S. and Katz, S. (2005). Concept mapping methodology: A catalyst for organizationl learning. *Evaluation and Program Planning*, 28, 257–269.

Thomas, P. M. and Altschuld, J. W. (1985). *Evaluators as Needs Assessment Consultants: An Application of the Delphi Technique to the Study of Education and Training Needs*. Paper presented at the joint meeting of the Canadian Evaluation Society, Evaluation Network and Evaluation Research Society: Toronto, ON.

Witkin, B. R. and Altschuld, J. W. (1995). *Planning and Conducting Needs Assessments*. Thousand Oaks, CA: Sage.

Clarificative Evaluation

10

Clarificative evaluation is designed to assist stakeholders to conceptualize interventions and improve their coherence, and thus increase the chances that their implementation will lead to desired outcomes. While responsibility for these actions would appear to be that of program developers, research shows that many developers have encountered difficulties in planning programs that they oversee (Bickman 2000).

This view resonates with our experiences in working with planners and policy managers across the government and not-for-profit sectors, and can be explained by factors such as:

- lack of time to fully research and articulate program plans;
- a preference to base practice on implicit or tacit understandings;
- the need to hurry implementation to meet political imperatives;
- increasing complexity in the nature of social interventions, particularly policy interventions that operate at different levels;
- multiple contributions by different departments or agencies towards a given policy; and
- increasing complexity and sophistication of program outcomes—for example, to meet 'triple bottom line' expectations of government.

Policy and program planning is often a complex activity. It is understandable that those responsible for interventions, many of whom have had little or no training in systematic planning procedures, have found planning tasks to be demanding.

The major product of Clarificative evaluation is a program plan that results from the collection and analysis of evidence. The use of inquiry is the feature that distinguishes Clarificative evaluation from conventional planning strategies.

Clarificative evaluation leads to better policy and program planning and explicit program designs. Over the past decade, interest in this Form of evaluation has burgeoned as agencies have looked for support to overcome barriers to more effective program provision.

Clarificative evaluation is concerned with:

- analysis and specification of the logic or theory of programs;
- establishing the feasibility of program design;
- encouraging consistency between program design and implementation; and
- providing a basis for program monitoring or impact evaluation.

Clarificative evaluation has a strong formative purpose and can be particularly useful when innovatory interventions are being planned and trialed. Normally, the evaluator works closely with program management and deliverers to conceptualize and describe the characteristics of the program and, in some cases, to provide validation of its quality.

Table 10.1 sets out the basic features of Clarificative evaluation in terms of the key dimensions of the Form.

KEY APPROACHES TO CLARIFICATIVE EVALUATION

The current importance of Clarification can be traced to developments in other Forms of evaluation practice. In the past, inadequacies in the specifications of many social and educational programs emerged when evaluators were asked to undertake traditional impact evaluations. Evaluators in these circumstances found that they were asked to evaluate 'non-events'—programs with little or no documentation. Sometimes programs had vague goals that provided little direction for those responsible for program delivery. From the point of view of evaluators undertaking impact evaluations, there was little or no basis for developing measures of implementation or outcomes.

From the early 1970s, Wholey (1983) and others, working as internal evaluators across federal government departments in the United States, developed procedures designed to overcome these deficiencies. These included strategies to improve the quality of program design to provide a firmer basis for subsequent impact evaluation. These efforts aimed to:

- identify the 'real' goals or intentions of a given program as distinct from the stated ones, as the basis for management of that program;
- identify unrealistic goals that were unachievable through the program and for which managers could not be held accountable;
- obtain consensus about goals held by different program providers;

Table 10.1 Summary of Clarificative evaluation

Dimension	Properties
Orientation	Clarification of program design including explication of program delivery
Typical issues	• What are the intended outcomes and how is the program designed to achieve them? • What is the underlying rationale for this program? • What program elements need to be modified in order to maximize the intended outcomes? • Is the program plausible? • Which aspects of this program are amenable to a subsequent monitoring or impact assessment?
State of program	Developmental
Major focus	All program elements
Timing (vis-à-vis program delivery)	Can be used to develop program *ab initio* but more likely to be during delivery, with particular relevance during early stages of program delivery
Key Approaches	• Evaluability assessment • Logic/theory development • Ex-ante
Assembly of evidence	Generally relies on combination of document analysis, interview and observation. Findings include program plan and implications for the organization. Process can lead to improved morale among program staff.

- elaborate the program through attention to how it worked in practice, as a way of making the program more plausible to policy-makers;
- identify various perceptions among managers and site-level providers about the program in an attempt to identify the underlying program logic.

An impact evaluation could not take place until the evaluator worked with program management to clarify what had been learnt in the design stage. The evaluator presented a model of the program: 'that portion of the program which is currently manageable in terms of a set of realistic program objectives and agreed on program performance indicators' (Wholey 1983). Thus the evaluator identified those aspects of the program that were amenable to rigorous evaluation designs for which 'measurable' data was available. Effectively this meant that aspects not amenable to measurement were not considered in the evaluation design.

Evaluability Assessment (EA)

Partly because of the emphasis on identifying measurable outcomes, an Approach now known as evaluability assessment, or EA, was developed (Rutman 1980). EA devotees have modified the outcomes emphasis towards a greater weight on design clarification as an end in its own right. There is now less emphasis on the clarification as a precursor to carrying out an impact evaluation. There has also been an orientation towards more involvement of stakeholders in the EA process.

The primary purposes of EA are to:

- refine program logic—that is, explication of the underlying cause and effect relationships, and functional aspects (resources and activities), with indicators as evidence for determining when planned activities are implemented and when intended and unintended outcomes are achieved; and
- identify stakeholders' awareness of and interest in a program—that is, their perceptions of what a program is meant to achieve, their concerns about program progress, perceptions of resource support and interests in evaluative information (for a variety of purposes). Stakeholders include all interested parties—for example, those providing resources, program managers and program deliverers.

There is a strong process element in EA designed to increase program commitment. Smith (1989b) reports that, after undertaking six major EAs in cooperative extension services, such as master gardening programs and water conservation studies,

> one of the changes from the original conceptualization of the process was the intense involvement of the program staff in every step. That change resulted in what I perceive as being one of the most important outcomes of the Cooperative Extension Services' EAs, *change in team member attitudes, knowledge and skills about evaluation and programming* (Smith 1989b: author's emphasis).

Smith goes on to note that, when a program is being planned, the first of the two purposes described above is the end point of the EA—that is, the outcome is a comprehensive program description. However, when the focus is an existing program, an effective EA will lead to an increased commitment to the implementation of the design. Policy-makers and program planners should thus be interested in evaluations that follow approaches suggested by Smith.

Program Logic (or Program Theory)

The construction and testing of program logic, or program theory, represents a second Approach to Clarificative evaluation. The terms 'logic' and 'theory' tend to be used interchangeably but in view of the increasing acceptance of the term 'evaluation theory' (see Shadish et al. 1991 as an example), we will use the term 'program logic' here. This serves to maintain a clear distinction between concepts that underlie current thinking about evaluation and program design respectively. According to Chen (1990), logic (theory) in this sense is defined as 'a set of interrelated assumptions, principles, and/or propositions to explain or guide social actions'.

Central to program logic is the nature of program causality, the ordering of events in such a way that the presence of one event or action leads to, or causes, a subsequent event or action. In programmatic terms, one could ask whether mechanism X causes outcome Y. While philosophers tell us that we can never be certain that X causes Y, it seems that unless we think in a causal fashion, there is no basis for developing interventions of any kind. Causal thinking is the fundamental basis for program planning.

The development of a means–ends hierarchy is an essential element of program logic. Patton (1997) and others have recommended the construction of a chain of objectives, implying the existence of actions whereby an objective at one level must be attained before the next can be accomplished. This notion of a program hierarchy is useful in that it largely does away with the confusion about outputs and outcomes that appears in some branches of the strategic planning literature.

Many theorists regard program logic as having two components:

- an explicit conceptualization of how the program causes the intended outcomes; and
- an evaluation that is based on this model (Rogers et al. 2000).

However, others see the development of the logic statement as an end in itself, in the same way that later proponents of EA have. For example, Patton (1997) says:

> At times, helping program staff or decision makers to articulate their programmatic theory of action is an end in itself. Evaluators are called

> on, not only to gather data, but also to assist in program design. Knowing how to turn a vague discussion of the presumed linkages between program activities and expected outcomes into a formal theory of action can be an important service to the program . . . On many occasions then, the evaluation data collection may include discovering and formalizing the program's theory of action (p. 162).

In such cases, Patton recommends that evaluators use techniques that are inductive, pragmatic and highly concrete. This is fundamental to the Clarificative Form of evaluation.

Likewise, Chen (1990) and his colleagues argue that evaluators should be engaged in the creation of a model of how a given program should work, the explication of the how and why. This involves recognition of crucial patterns and the development of a comprehensive framework in which these patterns are included. Chen distinguishes between two phases of evaluator action: normative and summative. In the normative phase, the program's logical structure is developed. In the summative phase, the model is tested in some way by empirical means.

In this chapter we are mostly concerned with the normative phase, in which the logic is developed and evaluators assist stakeholders in identifying, clarifying or developing goals or outcomes. 'Causal theory specifies the underlying causal mechanisms which link, mediate or condition the causal relationship between the treatment variable(s) and outcome variable(s) in a program' (Chen 1990).

One immediate source of evidence is documentation about the program, such as written information about the program plan. In addition, stakeholders, such as the program managers, can provide their views about assumptions and expectations. The evaluator constructs a tentative model in which any discrepancies are highlighted and, once these are resolved, a program model is produced. Thus there are similarities with EA and with Patton's (1997) methods described above.

But Chen (1990) departs from the high reliance on stakeholders' views because he maintains that they may not enable the clearest articulation of the complexity of the program's causal links. Chen likes to use social science theory to bolster information collected from stakeholders. This means gathering what is already known about the social or educational phenomenon under review. This is the use of the research review Approach within the Proactive Form, and is an illustration of how different Approaches can be used in conjunction. An example would be to review the literature on staff development to ensure that a given training program is well grounded, in addition to consulting with the program providers to take account of characteristics of the setting in the program design. Thus the evaluator brings his or her training and knowledge of the relevant research base to bear on the problem and constructs a model based on several sources.

For some evaluators, such as Pawson and Tilley (1998), reliance on social science theory is attractive in itself; however, in practice, we see the combination of information from research reviews and from stakeholders—particularly those actually providing the program—as most effective.

Weiss (1996) undertook a review of the use of program logic in evaluation practice. She makes an interesting distinction between program delivery and mechanisms that intervene between program delivery and the attainment of outcomes. These mechanisms are the responses to program delivery. She cites an example of a contraceptive counseling service:

> If contraceptive counseling is associated with reduction in pregnancy, the cause of the change might seem to be the counseling. But the mechanism isn't the counseling; that is the program activity, the program process. A common assumption would be that the mechanism is the knowledge that the counseling provides. But knowledge might not be the operating mechanism. It might be that the existence of the counseling program helps to overcome cultural taboos against family planning; it might give women confidence and bolster their assertiveness in sexual relationships; it might trigger a shift in the power relationships between men and women. These or any of several other cognitive/affective/social responses would be the mechanisms leading to the desired outcomes (p. 9).

Weiss makes the important point that full explication of a program should involve program logic in terms of mechanisms and details about delivery—how the program is to be implemented. She describes evaluations that include both as *theories of change (TOC) evaluations*. It should be noted that in program clarification we are concerned with implementation as much as with mechanisms expressed in one way or another, which is consistent with the Weiss view. Clearly some of these mechanisms must reside within the implementation and some in the ways in which participants react to the implementation process. This is a rich area for further evaluation research.

Funnell (2000) has extensive experience in program logic development. Working closely with program providers, she favors matrix formats that are based on a hierarchy of outcomes. For each outcome, the matrix includes:

- success criteria;
- program factors affecting success;
- non-program factors affecting success;
- activities and resources;

- performance information; and
- sources of data for determining performance.

The matrix thus contains both program development and monitoring components. Given that these matrices are tools for management, development and monitoring aspects are strongly interlinked. In this case, one could regard explication of the monitoring aspects as essential to the clarification exercise.

Example 10.1 Identifying important components and gaps in programs

Program clarification can be useful for clarifying new programs and including those not involved in tangible service delivery. Funnell's program logic Approach was used with an organization that promotes standards-based school reform at the state and national levels. An evaluation team, working with senior management, developed a framework which included ultimate intended outcomes of the program, how the program's activities were intended to lead to them, and the important intermediate outcomes. In addition, the evaluation team identified factors which could influence the achievement of each outcome, and what the program was currently doing to achieve them. This analysis helped the program administrators to identify gaps in their program logic and to recognize the importance of particular program activities (Rogers & Huebner 1998).

A second example of sophisticated program logic is found in the 'temporal logic model' (Den Heyer 2001), in which a series of logic frames is developed, for different stages of program implementation. One is prepared for the program planning stage, a second for the 'early' implementation stage, and so on. Each stage frame includes a column for modifications. Program staff are encouraged to use the findings from one stage to refine the next one. Proponents of this model believe that the monitoring process encourages informed decision-making as the program is rolled out, and the use of aggregated records to capture intended and unintended outcomes.

The work of Funnell and Den Heyer can be seen as a reaction to the limitations of the Logical Framework Analysis (the LogFrame), which has been widely used in international development programs supported by agencies such as the US Agency for International Development (USAID).

The purpose of the LogFrame is to delineate a program's elements and how they fit together. LogFrame is also used to report the success of the program against predetermined goals. The LogFrame is a matrix based on the following elements:

- goals;
- purpose;
- inputs; and
- outputs.

For each of these elements, a report is required on program characteristics, verifiable indicators, and sources of data for these indicators. A major criticism of the LogFrame is that it cannot inform implementation decisions as the program proceeds. Experience suggests that the LogFrame is used by international development agencies as a basic accountability mechanism, often requiring the attachment of minimal empirical evidence. Under these circumstances it is understandable that agencies responsible for delivering international aid programs have sought to develop alternative evaluation strategies. These are designed to meet the needs of other stakeholders, including the governments of countries where these programs are located, and providers and participants interested in program improvement.

Ex-ante evaluation

A third Approach within this Form is ex-ante evaluation. An ex-ante evaluation is an investigation which is undertaken in order to estimate and judge the impact of a future situation. This involves an assessment of the validity of a program's foundations, objectives and assumptions. It is thus necessary for these features to be clarified and subjected to tests of feasibility. Studies like this are increasingly being commissioned by government agencies before they commit themselves to program funding (Department of Justice 2004).

Examples of ex-ante evaluations draw on previous research and practice, and the substantive expertise of the evaluator. Some studies involve modeling—for example, to predict future economic costs and benefits (Roper et al. 2003). In the international development arena, a case has been made for the increased use of ex-ante evaluations in order to assure the outcomes of proposed expensive aid programs before they are commenced. However, Psacharopoulos (1995) notes the lack of use of ex-ante evaluations to guide decision-making in this arena. There is obviously a place for more research to be carried out on ways in which this Approach can be used, and the methods used to be integrated into other Approaches in the Clarificative Form.

CLARIFICATIVE EVALUATION: TRENDS AND CASE STUDIES

Assembling evidence

Table 10.1 includes a summary of ways in which evidence can be assembled within a Clarificative evaluation. There is high reliance on the collection of information that will assist the evaluator to construct a plausible program plan and to portray findings in ways that are readily understood by program managers and deliverers. Major sources of information are documentation, interviews and observations. Visits to the program site(s) are highly desirable.

Clarificative evaluation studies should:

- take into account the principles that have been developed in this chapter;
- involve the evaluator in a creative exercise involving the synthesis of information from a range of sources; and
- always produce an articulated program plan, usually presented in a schematic format.

A comprehensive guide to clarifying the essential features of a program has been provided by Smith (1989b). To use the Evaluability Assessment Approach she includes the following steps:

1 *Determine purpose, secure commitment, and identify evaluation team members*
An evaluator with experience in EA should be a key member of the evaluation task team that should be composed of members of the organization responsible for the program. Time is needed for the evaluation team to commit themselves to the program. A key task of the evaluation team is to identify the stakeholders and key influential decision-makers. Then the team needs to meet stakeholders and other influentials to explain the EA process.

2 *Define evaluation boundaries of program to be studied*
There is no hard and fast rule for defining the boundaries of the program. Smith suggests two factors should be taken into account: the importance of the program and decisions likely to be made. EAs should only be undertaken on a major program, not an isolated one-day event. Similarly, evaluators may need to ask decision-makers how an EA would be useful in decision-making before they decide to put resources into the evaluation effort. If the findings are not likely to make a difference, the EA should not be undertaken.

3 *Identify and analyze program documents*
Document analysis is central to the EA process. This includes legislation, hearings, debates, reports, policy statements, memoranda, research syntheses, program guidelines and resource statements. Smith counsels to read documents with care.

Conflicting documentary statements regarding what is intended and what is being accomplished may point to confusion among program personnel who read these documents and those who produce them. Two other suggestions are:

(a) note the purpose of each document: publicity handouts may contain mostly rhetoric whereas internal materials probably deal more with reality, albeit political; and
(b) identify quoted notes so that documents can be referenced and located later on.

4 *Develop and clarify program theory*
The approach is to develop a model closest to that which mirrors the reality of the implementation. Essentially, the exercise is the identification of the most critical, and to some extent general, elements of the program. Extensive consultation is necessary between members of the evaluation team and key program staff. Involving those who have a close working knowledge of what the program is like in the field, and representing different levels of implementation, best completes the exercise. Smith (1989b) notes that program staff who form part of the evaluation team are those most likely to benefit from developing the theory, and thus it is important that they be involved as much as possible in the exercise. Once the model has been developed, it should be returned to selected program staff for validation.

5 *Identify and interview stakeholders and describe their perceptions of the program*

6 *Identify stakeholders' needs, concerns and differences in perceptions*
Here the aim is to collect information concerning knowledge and opinions about the program from the stakeholders. The major aim is to identify the levels of awareness of and interest in the program. Information is generally collected by interviews and the usual canons of data collection, and analysis related to interviews applies. The key issues in these sections are to compare stakeholders' perceptions of the program with the program model, to validate any differences with more data, and to present an interim report on the findings to the primary client and other stakeholders.

7 *Determine plausibility of program model*
Plausibility is defined as the existence of necessary and sufficient conditions for a program to succeed. Components of a successful program are:

(a) a clear intention to bring about outcomes in participants;
(b) activities sufficient in quality and quantity to bring about the expected outcomes; and
(c) sufficient resources to implement these activities.

Judgments of program staff and other stakeholders should be used to work towards a plausible program. Interviews and group meetings are vehicles for determining whether the above conditions apply. When the goal of the EA is to plan a program, the question is one of intent; when the program is in action, the EA is used to work towards a plausibility of action.

8 *Draw conclusions and make recommendations*
Smith notes that conclusions are made throughout the EA, and that generally clients want recommendations to be made. As with all evaluations, she recommends that conclusions should be drawn with the best possible backup information.

9 *Plan specific uses for utilization of findings of the study*
Five possible decisions are possible. These are to decide whether to:

(a) stop the program, if it has not yet been implemented;
(b) change the program, if it has been implemented;
(c) undertake an outcomes evaluation, if the program as implemented is faithful to the refined program plan;
(d) take no further action; or
(e) take no notice of the findings of the EA.

It is the responsibility of the evaluator to come up with the product, on the basis of the evidence that has been assembled and analyzed. Coming up with a plausible program plan, whether it is in the form of a flow diagram, program logic or a written description, requires a combination of analytical and developmental data management skills.

Products of Clarificative evaluation

Fundamental to Clarificative evaluation is the portrayal of the design or plan of the program under review. It is up to the evaluator, in conjunction with the clients, to determine ways in which the design will be reported. A variety of formats exist, ranging from Boolean diagrams to extensive prose descriptions. The evaluator is encouraged to be creative in the use of these formats. Some examples follow.

Line diagrams

Clients may require only a rough conceptualization of a program as a line diagram, as shown in Example 10.2.

Example 10.2 The Job and Course Explorer (JAC) program

Job and Course Explorer (JAC) was a program designed to provide advice to young people about jobs and further study after secondary school. A major feature of JAC is a comprehensive data base of jobs and post-school courses. One aim of an evaluation of JAC was to identify the program logic of the JAC program as it had evolved over time. A round of visits to schools and employment agencies suggested that JAC in practice operated in the following ways:

a. central policy development and resource production

b.	counseling	curriculum use	'general'
	↓	↓	↓
c.	knowledge about courses and jobs	more effective and relevant curriculum	increased opportunities to use a computer
	↓	↓	↓

d. increased linkage between formal secondary education and requirements of the labor market and further education

A primary goal was to outline how a policy was being implemented at different site types (libraries, schools, prisons, etc.). The evaluation not only developed a conceptual model of implementation, but also described the relative importance of the major arms or activities, and assessed their effectiveness in achieving the overall goals of the JAC initiative. The development of what became the beginnings of a program logic arose from visits to sites. The approach is consistent with the development of a grounded theory (Glaser & Strauss 1967), and the use of investigatory methods of data management (Smith 1992).

Flow diagrams

Many studies include flow diagrams in their reports, using them as a basis for discussion. Figure 10.1 outlines a program logic as a series of if/then statements, used as the basis for planning the development of a water conservation program (Smith 1989a).

Figure 10.2 describes the logic of a rehabilitation intervention for people who incurred serious head injuries as a result of road trauma. Batterham (1991) developed the logic to assist management and staff providing the service to clarify the program plan, regarded as innovatory in rehabilitation care. Some of the model linkages highlight the more innovative approaches to rehabilitation, with those in the middle blocks representing support, autonomy and community-building.

Batterham remarks that:

> this model assumes that many head injured people can run up against a wall of behavioral and self-image problems that slow or halt functional progress. Traditional rehabilitation approaches would have abandoned these patients when progress halted due to these problems (p.11).

Objectives hierarchies

Another way in which a program can be represented is through an objectives hierarchy. As discussed earlier, a hierarchy represents a chain of objectives (or outcomes) in such a way that any one objective in the chain is the outcome of the attainment of the previous objective and, in turn, needs to be attained before the next objective in the hierarchy can be reached.

Example 10.3 depicts an innovative school curriculum based on individual student use of notebook computers in the classroom. This curriculum was introduced as a pilot at Year 5, for students about ten years of age, before being considered for use more widely across the school. Note that in addition to the objectives, Example 10.3 contains a set of underlying assumptions. One can think of them as providing a rationale for the relevance of each objective.

In this study, evaluators were invited into the school where the expectation was that they would perform an impact evaluation of the notebook program. However, as in many similar situations, it became clear that there was a need to first conceptualize the program, rather than to be concerned, at an early stage of implementation, with student outcomes. This objectives hierarchy was developed and reported to the school. This provided explicit direction for the implementation of the notebook curriculum over the next three years across other grade levels, and a framework by which the curriculum could be monitored.

Figure 10.1 Program logic for a water conservation program

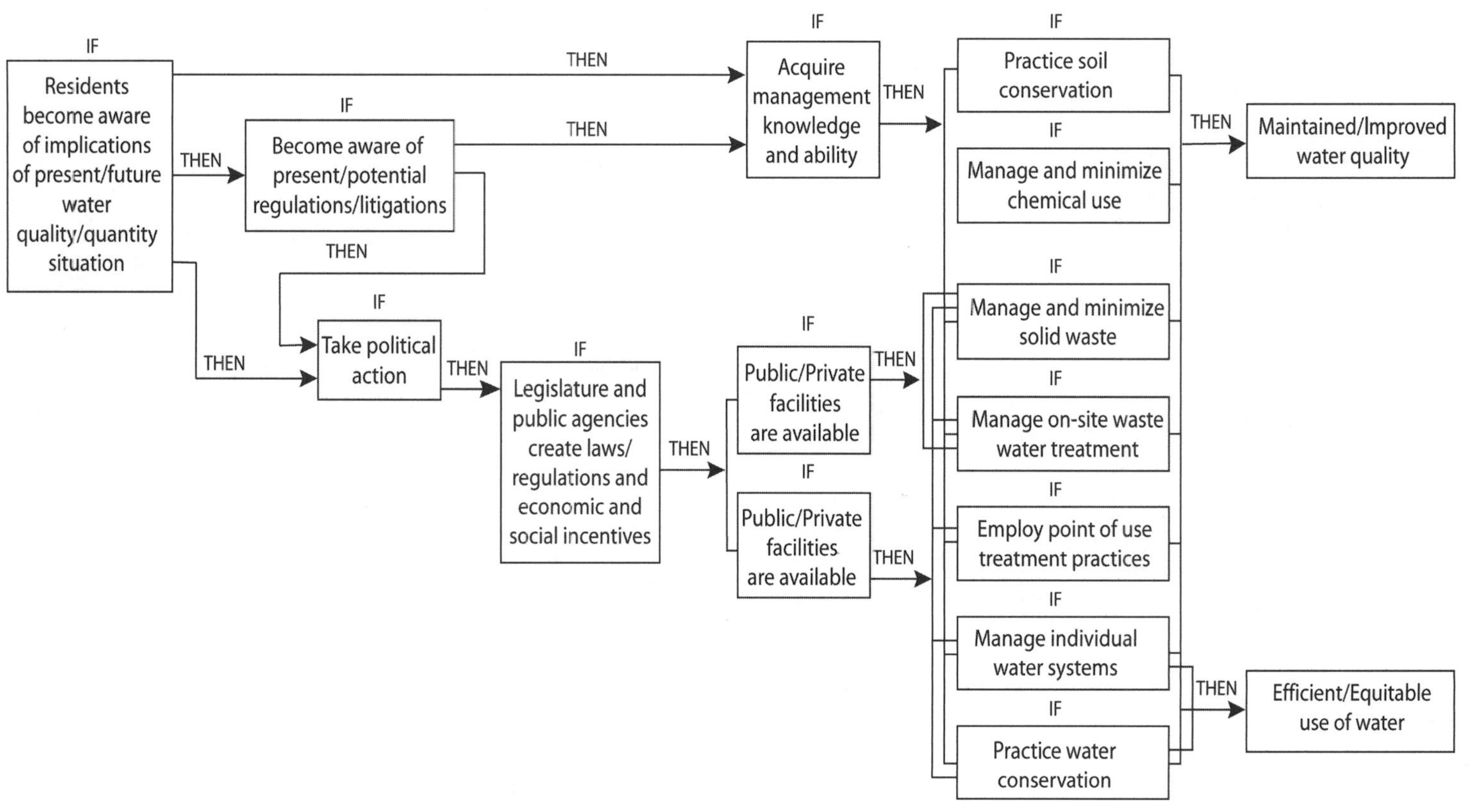

Figure 10.2 Program logic for an innovatory rehabilitation program

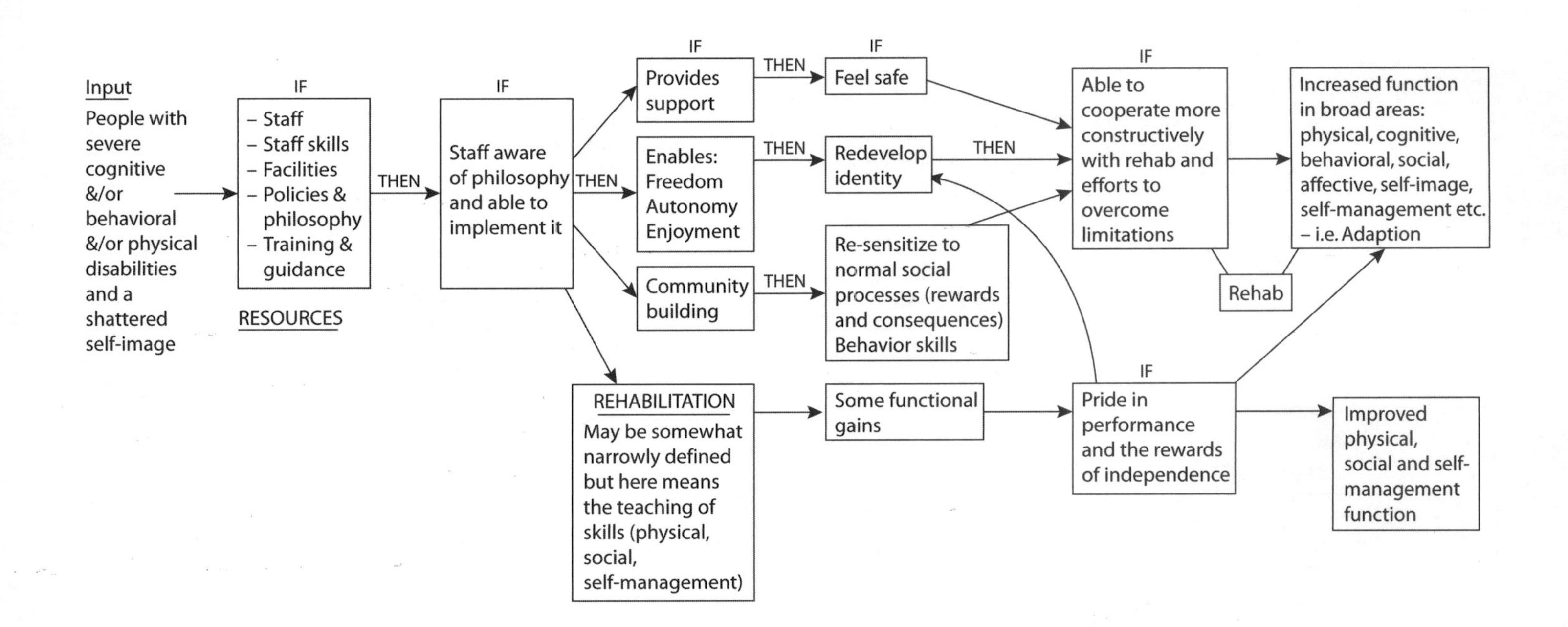

Example 10.3 An objectives hierarchy for the notebook computer initiative

Hierarchy of objectives	Underlying assumptions
III. Ultimate objectives	
15. To enhance students' ability to participate and contribute in a rapidly changing technological world.	Individuals who can participate in and contribute positively to the society at large will have a greater sense of personal control and lead more fulfilling lives.
14. To create a more rewarding teaching/learning environment.	Computer use enhances the quality of the classroom teaching/learning environment.
13. To integrate notebook computer use into the curriculum (i.e., to create a notebook curriculum).	Learning opportunities will be enhanced if computer use is integrated into the curriculum, not just regarded as a specialist, 'add on' skill remote from daily work.
12. To enhance awareness of the capability of computer technology.	All students require computer skills. (For girls in particular, it is important to learn to use the computer as a tool at an early age, and preferably to secondary school level.)
II. Intermediate objectives	
11. To provide more opportunities for students to learn independently at their own pace using their own learning materials.	Teachers should adopt a constructivist approach to curriculum, one where some of the knowledge is built by the learner, so not all is supplied by the teacher.
10. To develop data manipulation/research skills that can be applied to their own learning.	Students require strong data manipulation/research skills in order to pursue their learning.

Hierarchy of objectives	Underlying assumptions
9. To enhance creative problem-solving skills.	A high level of proficiency in programming is required to develop higher-order problem-solving skills.
8. To develop a strong level of proficiency in programming.	
I. Immediate objectives	
7. To increase the level of cooperation between students (in particular the propensity of more able students to work with others of less ability).	The portability of computers combined with the printed word facilitates and promotes a high level of interaction between students.
6. To enhance the acquisition of skills in literacy, word processing, and creative writing.	The ability to edit, to present work more clearly and to reflectively share written work via computer screens and classroom monitors enhances basic literacy and creative writing skills.
5. To develop skills of instructing and controlling the computer (e.g., basic programming).	The ability and willingness to apply the computer to learning situations depends upon level of keyboarding and programming skill.
4. To develop proficiency in basic keyboarding skills.	Proficiency in keyboarding, and in particular touchtyping skills, is fundamental to efficient computer use. Bad habits developed in poor initial training are difficult to rectify later.
3. To inform students about how to care for the computer, and the rules for handling/storage of computers and related hardware.	Rules and procedures for handling hardware and software in the classroom are fundamental to effective and efficient use.

Hierarchy of objectives	Underlying assumptions
2. To provide teachers with an understanding of how notebook computers and related software can be used to enhance the curriculum in core subjects (English, Humanities, Science and Math).	Beyond personal mastery of the hardware and software, teachers need to learn how to integrate the innovation into classroom practice to enhance learning.
1. To provide teachers with the basic skills related to personal mastery of the notebook computer and related hardware.	Personal mastery of the technology by teachers is a necessary prerequisite to successful introduction into the classroom.

Source: Owen, J. M. & Lambert, F. C. (1995) *Evaluation*, 1(2), 237–50.

In this evaluation, a flow diagram was also constructed, and is presented as Figure 10.3. Writing about this study, we said:

> [Figure 10.3] identifies the full range of program consequences and, in addition, places the program within the context of the total school system. Comparisons between this information and program documentation showed that the school had failed, in its initial planning, to anticipate the consequences of the program for: work that was already being done in specialist computer classes which continued during the trial; existing methods of student assessment and reporting which were standardized for Years 5, 6 and 7; and communication between teachers from different campuses (Owen & Lambert 1995).

Inclusions of implications for the school as a whole appear in the lower part of Figure 10.3. These implications are consistent with a more general research finding—that the introduction of an innovation into an organization has implications for the organization as a whole, and that evaluators should be sensitive to this fact. Merely providing findings about the program without attending to organizational consequences often leaves decision-makers with less than a satisfactory level of information about what action to take.

Descriptive product

While most program logic findings are presented in schematic style, a descriptive format is also acceptable (see Example 10.4).

Figure 10.3 Program logic statement informed by the evaluation: adding a systems perspective

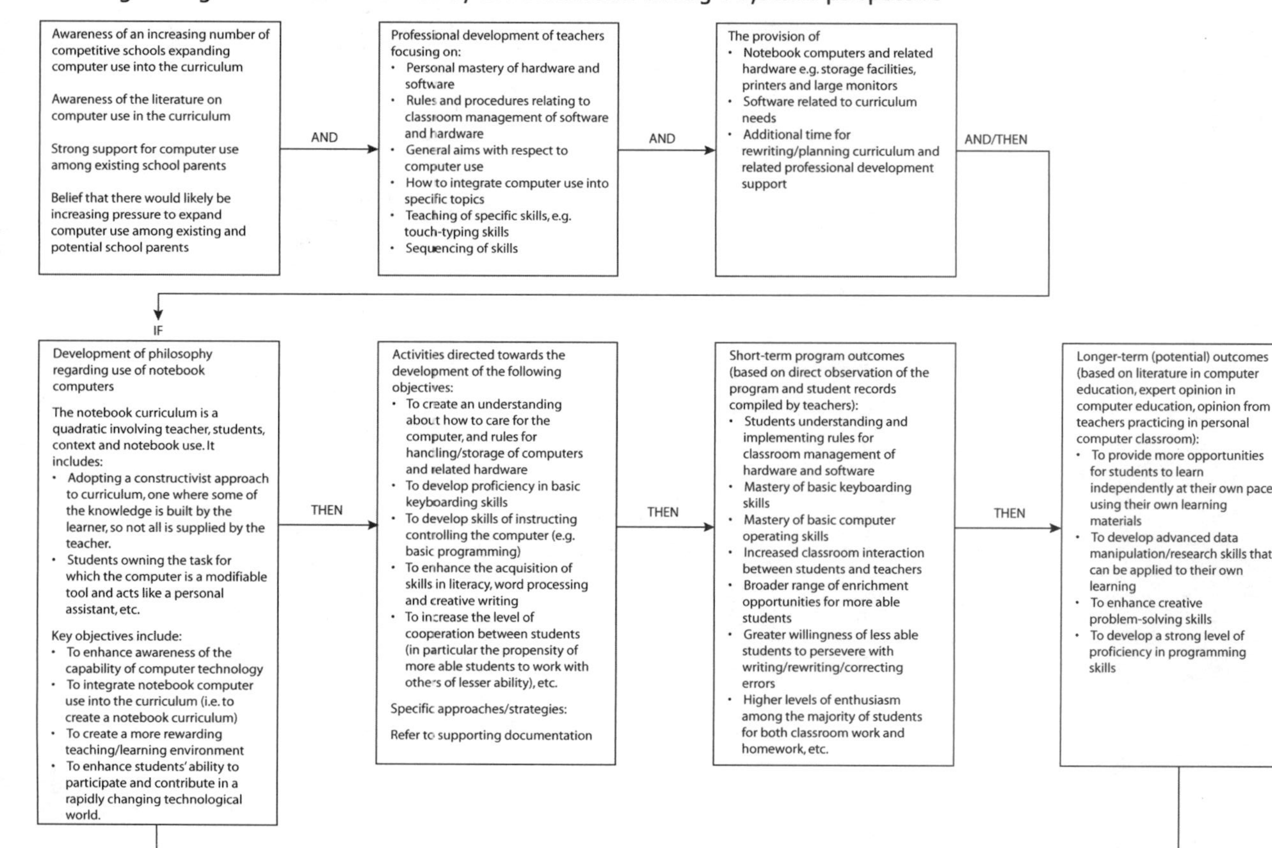

BUT

Unintended outcomes:

- Inadequate levels of proficiency in touch-typing/keyboarding skills in both students and teachers
- Parts of the normal curriculum being omitted, not teaching to standard Year 5 curriculum content
- Overlap/confusion/inconsistencies between work covered in separate computer classes and computer work done in home-room classes in core subjects
- Lack of relevance of existing forms of student assessment and reporting
- Excessive stress levels among home-room teachers, and a perception that program deliverers were not able to influence the decisions made about the program
- Disillusionment with the Technology Working Party as the coordinating body for the program
- Resentment between campuses, inadequate coordination sharing of resources, etc.

Implications for the total school scheme

Broader curriculum implications:

- How and when should keyboarding be introduced to students? (i.e. is Year 5 the most appropriate year for this basic skill building?)
- What is the rationale for continuing to offer separate specialist computer classes at the Year 5 level? If they are continued, what should the content be?
- If continuity of classroom experience is important for mastering basic computer operating skills, what changes might avoid Year 5 classroom being a floating population in the introductory stages of computer use (i.e. implications for time-tabling music and sport, remedial instruction, enrichment, etc.)
- Given the different skills and content embodied in the notebook computer curriculum, what methods of student assessment and reporting are most suitable? How will these relate to the reporting at other levels?

Implications for professional development and support:

- Should teachers receive more hands-on experience with hardware and software before tackling the program in the classroom?
- In light of the double burden this innovation imposes, what additional types of support can be given to teachers? What changes in institutional structure are necessary to ensure this support is there when needed?

Implications for institutional structures:

- How effective is the Technology Working Party and its current mode of operation in responding to the implementation demands of the program? Would alternative institutional arrangements be more responsive to the needs of teachers?
- Should a projects officer be given responsibility for the daily management and coordination of the program, and a small subcommittee formed to report to the Technology Working Party on matters relating to the notebook curriculum and resources required for its implementation?

Example 10.4 Development of principles of Enterprise Education

The Country Education Project (CEP) is an agency designed to improve the quality of education in rural areas. Heavily committed to community participation, the CEP has a history of encouraging innovative programs in schools and in the small communities serviced by the schools.

One initiative was to provide seeding for the development of Student Enterprise programs in a small number (about ten) of the 300 individual rural schools across the state. These programs involved students planning and implementing small business ventures as part of the curriculum in the middle years of secondary school (Years 9–10).

Towards the end of the first year of operation of these trial programs, an evaluation was commenced which aimed to develop documentation on Enterprise Education. The purpose of the evaluation was to synthesize Enterprise Education principles and a program plan from the practice of these innovatory programs.

The plan could then be used as a basis for the adoption and implementation of Enterprise Education in rural schools which were not participants in the trial phases to develop their own programs.

An evaluation team followed many of the principles suggested by Smith (1989b). In addition to analysis of documentation, visits were made to the sites where Enterprise Education was trialed. Teachers, community representatives and students were interviewed. In addition, a literature search was undertaken.

The evaluators drew up some tentative principles of Enterprise Education which were synthesized from the best of the innovative practice. Key players, teachers and representatives of the CEP executive were asked to comment on the developed principles. As a result of these procedures, a final plan was developed. The plan was organized around seven elements of Enterprise Education:

1 Selection of a team and working together;
2 Creative thinking;
3 Planning the enterprise;
4 Getting underway;
5 Implementing the plan;
6 Monitoring procedures; and
7 Modifying procedures.

In addition, the evaluation identified issues associated with the successful introduction of Enterprise Education into a rural secondary school. These included the following:

- Student Enterprise should not be seen as an 'extra', outside the mainstream of school curriculum. Enterprise projects to become embedded in the school curriculum need:
  - strong commitment on the part of teachers and school principals;
  - cooperation with the local community, and initiative and entrepreneurship in developing and sustaining programs;
  - continuous evaluation leading to ongoing staff development and adaptation to student needs;
  - significant departures from traditional schooling in response to individual student needs in a pluralistic society.
- The implementation of Student Enterprise projects requires a shift in pedagogy, from an emphasis on directed teaching to one of enabling students to learn. At the same time, teachers must be clear about the skills students will acquire. A review of Enterprise programs concluded that: 'A great deal of present practice in what might be termed enterprise skill development is not accountable for the skill formation of learners. Too many workers with young people . . . focus on broad generalities such as personal development, self esteem and empowerment and do not pay enough attention to identifying skills and discussing their relevance to the personal and career objectives of the young people'.
- There is a fine line between too much assistance and too little help from teachers and others. On the one hand, Enterprise Education is designed to foster self initiative, and thus it is inappropriate for teachers to use 'lock-step' approaches. On the other hand, there is no doubt that teachers need to set up structures to facilitate the processes. Without them, projects can flounder. At least one CEP project almost came to grief due to lack of assistance at crucial times in its implementation.
- Enterprise skill development should not be seen as the only way of organizing learning. However, it is an important strategy for preparing students for the realities engendered by a rapidly changing society and associated employment conditions.
- Most students carrying out a CEP Enterprise project found that it was harder than they had expected. More that one team reported that the project was 'not as easy as we thought

it would be'. It is clear that Enterprise projects were no soft option, requiring intellectual and other skills at least on a par with more traditional school subject work.

- School-level evaluations showed that learning management and organizational skills were major outcomes of the innovatory projects. These included: time management, teamwork, communication, problem-solving, budgeting and marketing, and working and negotiating with a range of people. It was through the acquisition of these skills that, at the conclusion of their projects, students had gained confidence and pride in their achievements.

Following the evaluation, a report was disseminated to all rural schools in the system. Knowing that the audience was principals who had no knowledge of program logic, we concluded that the most effective means of reporting would be to prepare a brochure using simple short-prose style. Thus no diagrams were used to outline the essential features of the program. The report included key elements of program design in prose form: objectives, implementation and rationale.

Mindful of the interaction between program innovation and organizational change mentioned above, we included a section titled 'Integrating Student Enterprise into the School Curriculum'. The outcome was a consolidated system-wide Program plan. This study is consistent with what Weiss (1996) has described as a 'theory of change' evaluation.

Another feature of this study was that the evaluators cooperated with policy developers in determining the style of reporting and with dissemination strategies (Owen & Andrew 1989). This example suggests a further use of Clarificative evaluation over those suggested by others—namely, the dissemination of the essential features of a program in a clarified state to a range of sites not yet using that program.

CONCLUSION

This chapter has outlined the bases for Clarificative evaluation and some key Approaches to practice consistent with the need to help make explicit the logic of programs.

It is important to reiterate that the evaluator is engaged in an investigation. Evidence must be collected and analyzed. A novel feature of this Form of evaluation, compared with other Forms, is that the product of the inquiry contains a fully developed and explicit program specification.

It is also important to note a likelihood that the Clarification Form will be used in conjunction with other evaluation Forms, a point made by recent commentators on developments in the use of the Program Logic Approach (Rogers et al. 2000).

Conceptually, the use of Clarificative Approaches should precede the use of Monitoring and Impact Forms. While Clarification provides the basis for monitoring and impact studies, one could argue that the use of the Clarification Form to assure the delivery of programs is of higher benefit to many providers and program clients. This view is consistent with the theme of this book, which is that evaluative inquiry should be seen as the servant of effective program provision.

There is no doubt that program managers and deliverers value having a sound basis for their programs. While program staff can sometimes develop a workable program design alone, an evaluator with strong analytical and creative skills can contribute to a program design that more accurately and comprehensively represents its intentions and implementation characteristics.

The knowledge base underlying Clarification evaluation has moved ahead since this area came to the attention of evaluation scholars (Bickman 1987), but challenges remain. For those with interests in policy evaluation, the management of multi-level logic model development and implementation needs to be addressed. This could provide a valuable contribution to the successful implementation of complex policy, for improvement and accountability purposes. We are only beginning to think about how evaluators can assist with these complex interventions.

REFERENCES

Batterham, R. (1991). *Are Clinical Indicators Bullies?* Unpublished paper for the Graduate Diploma in Evaluation, The University of Melbourne.

Bickman, L. (1987). Barriers to the use of program theory. *Evaluation and Program Planning*, 12(4), 387–390.

Bickman, L. (2000). Summing up program theory. *New Directions for Evaluation*, 87, 103–112.

Chen, H. (1990). *Theory Driven Evaluation*. Newbury Park: Sage.

Den Heyer, M. (2001). *The Temporal Logic Model*. Ottawa, Canada: International Development Research Centre.

Department of Justice (2004). *Feasibility Study: Resource Tracking and Information Management System*. Melbourne, Victoria: Victorian Government, Department of Justice.

Funnell, S. C. (2000). Developing and using a program theory matrix for program evaluation and performance monitoring. *New Directions for Evaluation*, 87, (Fall), 91–102.

Glaser, B. and Strauss, A. L. (1967). *The Discovery of Grounded Theory.*

Chicago, IL: Aldine.
Owen, J. M. and Andrew, P. F. (1989). *Student Enterprises: Learning by Doing*. Melbourne: Centre for Program Evaluation, The University of Melbourne, for the Country Education Project.
Owen, J. M. and Lambert, F. C. (1995). Roles for evaluation in learning organizations. *Evaluation*, 1(2), 259–73.
Patton, M. Q. (1997). *Utilization Focused Evaluation*. 3rd ed. Thousand Oaks, CA: Sage.
Pawson, R. and Tilley, N. (1998). *Realistic Evaluation*. London: Sage.
Psacharopoulos, G. (1995). Using evaluation indicators to track the performance of education programs. *New Directions for Evaluation*, 67 (Fall), 93–104.
Rogers, P. J. and Huebner, T. A. (1998). *Using Program Theory for Organizational Learning and Formative Evaluation*. Paper given at the annual conference of the Canadian Evaluation Society: St Johns, Newfoundland.
Rogers, P. J., Petrosino, A., Huebner, T. A. and Hacsi, T. A. (2000). Program theory evaluation: Practice, promise, and problems. *New Directions for Evaluation*, 87, (Fall), 5–13.
Roper, S., Hewitt-Dundas, N. and Love, J. H. (2003). An ex-ante evaluation framework for the regional benefits of publicly supported R&D projects. *Research Policy*, 33(3), 487–509.
Rutman, L. (1980). *Planning Useful Evaluations*. Beverly Hills, CA: Sage.
Shadish, W. R., Cook, T. D. & Leviton, L. C. (1991). *Foundations of Program Evaluation*. Newbury Park: Sage.
Smith, M. F. (1989a). 'Evaluability Assessment of the Maryland Water Quality/Quantity Program'. Personal communication.
Smith, M. F. (1989b). *Evaluability Assessment: A Practical Approach*. Norwell, MA: Kluwer.
Smith, N. L. (1992). 'Aspects of investigative inquiry in evaluation'. *New Directions for Program Evaluation*, 56, 3–13.
Weiss, C. H. (1996). *Theory Based Evaluation: Past, Present and Future*. Paper presented at the annual meeting of the American Evaluation Association, Atlanta, CA.
Wholey, J. (1983). *Evaluation and Effective Public Management*. Boston, MA: Little, Brown.

Interactive Evaluation

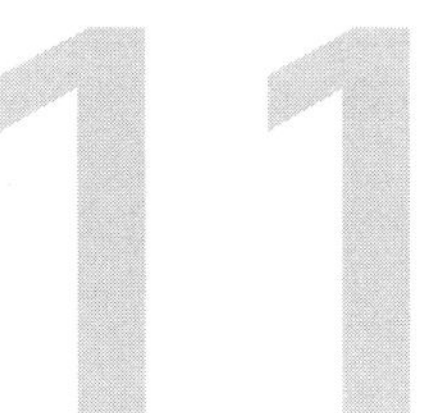

The control of providers over program development and delivery is fundamental to *Interactive* (or Participatory) *evaluation*. The evaluator provides input and support for the agenda of organizations, providers and community groups. Evaluation efforts are internal, influenced strongly by those who are 'close to the action', and evaluators employ interactive strategies to encourage utilization of findings (Huberman & Cox 1990). Evaluation is seen as one input that contributes to the working knowledge of individuals and organizations, supplementing existing craft knowledge and knowledge about the local context (Owen 2003).

Over the past decade, Interactive evaluation has become a 'hot topic', fueled by the interests of theorists about possibilities and benefits. In addition to the mainstream, Interactive evaluation has been championed by agencies not previously associated with internal evaluation, such as the World Bank, in the context of international aid and development. However, despite some interesting contributions (for example, Karlsson Vestman 2004), empirically based case studies of organizational benefits are difficult to find in the literature.

Interactive evaluation is concerned with:

- the provision of systematic evaluation findings through which local providers can make decisions about the future direction of their programs;
- providing assistance in planning and carrying out self-evaluations;
- focusing evaluation on organizational change and improvement, in most cases on a continuous basis; and
- a perspective that evaluation can be an end in itself, as a means of empowering providers and participants.

Table 11.1 Summary of Interactive evaluation

Dimension	Properties
Orientation	Improvement of program already being delivered
Typical issues	• What is this program trying to achieve? • How is this service going? • Is the delivery working? • Is delivery consistent with the program plan? • How could delivery be changed to make it more effective? • How could this organization be changed to make it more effective?
State of program	Under initial implementation, or subject to continuous review and improvement
Major focus	Major focus is on delivery but findings could influence changes in program plan and thus affect outcomes
Timing (vis-à-vis program delivery)	During delivery
Key Approaches	• Responsive • Action research • Developmental • Empowerment • Quality review
Assembly of evidence	Relies on intensive onsite study, including observation and interview. Extent to which data collection is systematic depends on Approach. Providers may also be involved in the evaluation to varying extents, from total responsibility to conclusion drawing.

Interactive evaluation has a strong formative purpose—that is, the findings are normally expected to contribute to organizational and program improvement.

Table 11.1 sets out the basic features of the Interactive Form.

Interactive evaluation can be linked to a framework of change within the Problem Solving Model (Havelock 1971). This model assumes that where those responsible for a given problem have the ability and inclination to deal with that problem. If outsiders are involved they are involved on the terms set by the providers. The model is thus predicated on the adequacy of local expertise to deal with local problems and to call for outside assistance when needed. In such a scenario, external knowledge—in particular, accumulated research-based knowledge—is of marginal relevance. External policies and directives do not play a major role in shaping program delivery and associated evaluative procedures.

Consistent with the problem-solving model is a view that each program initiative is 'new'—that is, it can be regarded as an innovation from the perspective of those involved in its delivery. Programs that are consistent with this view:

- attempt to address problems that have not been subject to program intervention before; or
- employ program structures or processes that are unique, at least from the point of view of the program staff.

Typically, organizational and program objectives are evolving rather than preordinate, sometimes not fully explicit, and thus open to debate. Those directly involved might expect to come to a steady state in terms of general direction over a period of time, but continue to reserve the right to use new or alternative strategies to achieve program goals—that is, there is ongoing adaptation and responsiveness.

Program delivery can be idiosyncratic and there is little, if any, regard for consistency of treatment, uniform implementation or outcomes. In some systems, there is government support for problem-solving, based at least partly on an ideological position that there should be local control over decisions that affect the local community.

Example 11.1 Landcare

A policy of local control has been adopted by a department of agriculture known as Landcare, which aims to reduce deleterious effects on the rural environment by encouraging farmers and others employed on the land to adopt programs that address local concerns. These include erosion due to excess land clearance, raising of the water table and increased salinity, and spread of noxious weeds. Rural communities are given limited resources to apply to problems that arise in their region. Devolution of responsibility of this nature has been found to be successful due in no small part to the commitment of local people, and the additional resources they bring to the program in terms of time, travel and use of their own materials, resources which would otherwise have to be provided by government.

Use of Interactive evaluation can be linked to the following aspects of organizational development:

1 *Organizational learning*. This is a continuous process of growth and improvement that:

- uses internal feedback about processes and outcomes to make changes;
- is integrated into work activities and within an organization's infrastructure (for example, culture, systems and structures, leadership and communication mechanisms); and
- seeks the alignment of values, attitudes and perceptions among organizational members (Garvin 1995; Torres 2001).

The assumption that organizations can learn by inquiry into practice reflects a broader need for continuous relevant knowledge for decision-making in social, political and economic spheres of endeavor in a civil society (Sowell 1996).

2 *Evaluation culture*. Based on a series of studies, we suggest that internal evaluation and evaluation culture are related in the following ways:

An internal evaluation regime is consistent with an organization becoming a center of inquiry. In such a regime, we no longer think of organizations simply as knowledge distribution centers. An organization must be concerned with more than delivery; it must also be a producer as well as a transmitter of knowledge. One can think of an organization with this perspective as engaged in a pervasive search for meaning it its work. If this position is adopted, then the organization has developed a culture of evaluation (Owen 2003, p. 44).

Key factors which affect the development of an evaluation culture include:

- roles of management: initiation and follow-through by operational managers, in-principle sanction by senior management, and linkage to and sustained support from timely external expertise where required; and
- effective change and innovation strategies: the use of an incremental approach to evaluation, disseminating information about evaluation to staff, early demonstration of rewards and benefits for staff, and 'neutralization' of opposition (Owen 2003, p. 47).

3 *Evaluation capacity building (ECB)*. This is defined as:

> a context dependent intentional action system of guided processes and practices for bringing about and sustaining a state of affairs in which quality program evaluation and its appropriate uses are ordinary and ongoing practices within or between one of more organizations/programs/sites (Stockdill et al. 2002, p. 8).

In simple terms, one could think of these related concepts forming a cause and effect chain. For example, if an organization sets out to build its evaluation capacity in ways that are consistent with effective change literature findings, an evaluation culture would emerge. The existence of an evaluation culture would, in turn, sustain the evaluation component of an organizational commitment to learning.

KEY APPROACHES TO INTERACTIVE EVALUATION

Attributes of well-known Approaches consistent with Interactive evaluation are outlined below.

Responsive evaluation

Stake (1980) is the theorist most associated with methodologies consistent with this Approach. An evaluation is responsive if:

- it orients more directly to program activities than to program intents;
- it responds to audience requirements for information;
- the value perspectives of program stakeholders are referred to in reporting the success and failure of the program.

Stake has used these principles to structure his fieldwork. It is noteworthy that he is an external evaluator: in problem-solving terms, he is an 'outsider'. He prefers to immerse himself at the evaluation site, negotiate the boundaries of the study, base data collection on observation, and write extensive case study reports. Interpretation and discussion of these reports, and other more informal means of reporting, are designed to help practitioners reach new understandings by placing their existing craft knowledge alongside the findings of the evaluation. This is referred to as 'naturalistic generalization'. Stake assumes that this will lead to improved practice. The instrumental use of Responsive evaluation has not been well documented, however, and we would value examples of how practitioners translate evaluation findings into practice. For other evaluators adopting this Approach, there are related questions. Does the evaluator help clients work through the implications of the case analysis? Does one provide summaries for those too busy to read an entire case report? Does the evaluator have the 'right' to indicate action implied by the findings of the study?

Stake's approach is orientated towards client understanding. This is a legitimate evaluation role (see Chapter 6), in that Responsive evaluation leads to enlightenment of stakeholders from which they can make decisions about program change. This Approach provides an illumination of issues that take into account knowledge of the context in which the program is set.

Action research

Action research is a second Approach used in the context of site-level improvement and local control. What is action research and how does it link to the needs of practitioners and, more generally, to Interactive evaluation? Action research had its beginnings in the search for local-level solutions to on-the-job problems. Lewin (1946) wrote about its use in areas such as race relations and community housing more than half a century ago.

Orton (1992) defines action research as:

> a collaborative research, centered in social practice, which follows a particular process, espouses the values of independence, equality and cooperation, and is intended to be a learning experience for those involved, to produce a change for the better in the practice and to add to social theory (p. 11).

Wadsworth (1991) views the process as a cyclic one involving the following components:

- *Reflection on current action*. Every now and then, site-level practitioners notice a discrepancy of action, between what they do or experience and what they expect to be happening.
- *Design*. Practitioners make explicit the problem and set out to answer questions which will assist with solving the problem. At this stage it is also important to identify whose problem it is. A critical reference group should be set up at this stage composed of those with a stake in the inquiry.
- *Fieldwork*. Emphasis here is placed on evidence collection to determine the meanings of the action from the perspective of each of the critical reference group members.

- *Analysis and conclusions*. The fieldwork allows the generation of insights that lead to understandings not previously thought of. There is an emphasis on understanding the meaning of the action. Conclusions, explanations and even theories are generated.
- *Planning*. It is now possible to consider changes and options for improved action. Imaginative but realistic recommendations can be made and put into practice. These are well grounded in past practice and the experience of learning from it.

A fundamental feature of action research is that it concentrates on evaluating implementation of a possible *solution* to a site-level problem. Kemmis (1985) describes four 'moments' of action research as follows:

- Develop a plan of action to improve what is already happening.
- Act to implement the plan.
- Observe the effects of action in the context of which it occurs.
- Reflect on these effects as a basis for further planning, subsequent action, and so on, through a succession of cycles.

Kemmis is specific about the order of these phases. The plan is constructed action and by definition it must be prospective and forward-looking. This can include a trial of innovatory practice that originates outside the immediate experience of the practitioner. For example, in a teaching situation, this could involve the introduction of group techniques where the practitioner has been accustomed to didactic styles of teaching. Consistent with the Interactive Form, an important aspect of action research is that the innovation is not imposed; it would be introduced on the basis of an expressed need of the practitioner. In an educational setting, for example, this could mean adopting teaching practices that are more conducive to elucidating the content matter or improving the learning of students. Others support this view. For example, Brown (1990) states:

> at the core of the notion of group self-evaluation lies the concept of action research; a recurrent cyclic approach to planning, action, observing the outcomes, reflecting on them and replanning on the basis of what has been understood. For those who engage in it, it provides the prospect of enhanced understanding leading to improved performance. It is essentially a simple idea and one that has a natural appeal for people in new circumstances or engaging in new activities (p. 1).

Wadsworth (1991) suggests a number of opportunities for developing a comprehensive program of group self-evaluation:

- *Daily informal personal reflection*. Good practitioners intuitively reflect on their teaching practices and modify them accordingly on a day-to-day basis.

- *Weekly reviews*. These might involve making special diary notes on the progress of particular students, reviewing the week's diary to reflect on priorities and time management issues, or arranging informal discussion time with colleagues to discuss facets of program operations.
- *Special-effort evaluations of particular aspects of practice*. These will be evaluations which respond to the immediate concerns of those involved in program activities. For example, there may be some concern that the program is not satisfactorily reaching those who need it most. This might prompt an investigation of current strategies for reaching the target group, and might in the initial stages lead to an evaluation of the program newsletter.
- *Monthly collective problem-pooling sessions*. Such sessions could provide a forum for raising new issues, identifying those issues clearly in need of action, or tabling contentious issues for further discussion and/or research.
- *Annual 'what-have-we-achieved?'* and *'where-are-we-heading next year?'* workshops. This might involve reports from individuals reflecting on the program over the year, brainstorming sessions about future program development and identifying action that needs to be taken.

In summary, there is a debate about where the cycle of Action Research begins. In work we have undertaken in the context of organizational improvement, the view adopted by Wadsworth has been preferred by practitioner groups. That is, there has been a tendency to first ask questions about the *current* situation with a view to deciding how this situation can be improved. For example, a trainer might wish to know how she spends her time in a typical staff development activity as the basis of deciding how to manage her time more effectively. Then, in a second stage, the trial of an innovation—say, a new method of time management—would be monitored. For the practitioner, this would be seen as a logical follow-up within the one review and improvement process.

Developmental evaluation

This Approach has been championed by Patton (1996) in the United States and Cousins and Earl (1992) in Canada and requires ongoing commitment from a key evaluation adviser.

The evaluator is part of a team whose members collaborate to conceptualize, design and test new interventions in a long-term ongoing process of continuous improvement, adaptation and intentional change. The evaluator's primary function with the team is to elucidate team discussions with evaluative questions, data and logic, and to facilitate evidence-based decision-making in the developmental process (Patton 1996).

Unlike Quality Review, discussed later in this chapter, the evaluator is constantly available for assistance with almost any aspect of concern to the organization. Compared with the Responsive Approach, the evaluator is likely to spend less time in data collection and analysis, and more time in assisting others to undertake these activities. Some see the role of the evaluator as akin to an organizational development consultant. We have argued earlier in this book that the roles of evaluator and supporter of organizational change are becoming fuzzier. Patton (1996) may be pointing the way to the future in which the evaluator profession will accept that the provision of timely advice to managers and program providers based on evaluation expertise, broadly rather than narrowly defined, will represent the new orthodoxy.

EMPOWERMENT EVALUATION

Of the Approaches associated with Interactive evaluation, Empowerment evaluation has attracted the most controversy. From the time when he was president of the American Evaluation Association (in 1993), Fetterman has disseminated principles of empowerment and their use as a basis for evaluation. Self-determination, defined as the ability to chart one's own course in life, is a basic tenet of Empowerment evaluation. Organizations and individuals must be able to find ways to bring relevant information to bear on problems and find solutions (Fetterman & Wandersman 2004).

Key tenets of empowerment are as follows:

- The most meaningful changes are those that occur in the people themselves, those that reflect an increased capacity for initiating and carrying out social change.
- The definition of human capacity is more concerned with self-sufficiency, self-determination and empowerment than with changes that can be statistically measured.
- Success is measured by the extent to which people are able to identify their own problems and form a consensus to propose appropriate solutions.
- Change occurs best when greater emphasis is placed on the process for change while maintaining a focus on the results of change (Dugan 1996).

Fetterman is just as concerned with the notion of empowerment as with the roles of evaluation (Fetterman et al. 1996). He suggests that, in practice, empowerment involves program staff, participants and evaluators in:

- collaborating to come to a consensus about their mission, vision and expected results;
- taking stock of what they already have and using this as a baseline to plan for the future; and
- using evaluation as a tool to develop strategies linked to the attainment of specific goals.

The Empowerment Approach:

- is designed to create a 'folk culture' of evaluation;
- is a mechanism used to create and drive a learning organization;
- is not mutually exclusive to more traditional Impact evaluation undertaken by external evaluators; and
- can be fostered by experienced evaluators through the following:
  - training others to acquire evaluation skills
  - acting as facilitators or coaches to help others conduct evaluation
  - undertaking illuminative evaluations in conjunction with practitioners, and
  - acting as advocates for disadvantaged groups (Fetterman 1994).

In practice, the role of the evaluator generally spans roles associated with program planning and delivery, in addition to those more often associated with evaluation practice. There is an implication that the evaluator will be committed to an organization for a period of time, during which there is an expectation that more of the major programmatic and evaluative decisions will pass to program staff and participants. The Empowerment Approach has also been described as Transformative Participatory Evaluation (Cousins & Whitmore 1998, p. 7).

Quality review (institutional self-study)

Quality reviews usually take place in individual agencies that are responsible for program delivery within systemic policy directives. Reviews would be the responsibility of, say, each manager in a chain of hotels, or the principal of each school within a school district. This Approach could also apply within one organization in which there are logical sub-groups—for example, to all wards in a large public hospital.

The major propositions which underlie the quality review are that:

- the system provides guidelines for self-evaluation and improvement;
- effective agency-level development is enhanced by the implementation of system-level guidelines to support local problem-solving; and
- all agencies are expected to undertake such processes within a given time span (Cuttance 1994).

In the most effective quality reviews, a selection of operations is identified for evaluation by each agency. These are the ones that would repay greatest return for further development. In doing so, agencies might address factors such as:

- those enabling current successful programs;
- those impeding current performance;
- areas of development necessary to meet emergent needs of clients in the future; and
- effectiveness of system-level services provided by the system to the agency.

It is generally assumed that program staff can undertake Quality reviews. They can be added to staff workloads without additional agency assistance except for staff training and the provision of manuals for guidance. Expertise in the form of experienced evaluators is generally not available. Experience in the use of Quality reviews suggests, however, that they tend to impose unrealistic burdens on staff, who are rarely in a position to refuse to cooperate. There is also usually a tension between an improvement-focused agency effort and a requirement to inform the system-level authority of the findings of the evaluation. Nevertheless, there are instances where agencies have grasped the autonomy to make changes and improvements based on the review process.

INTERACTIVE EVALUATION: TRENDS AND CASE EXAMPLES

Interactive evaluation practitioners often borrow principles and concepts from across the major Approaches. In this section we present a range of examples that are consistent with good practice.

Response to client agendas

Evaluators are expected to respond to the concerns of clients in evaluation. However, in Interactive evaluation, the evaluator should be especially attuned to the needs of clients, and adopt a close 'psychological proximity' in dealing with all aspects of the evaluation process.

Example 11.2 Country Education Project

The Country Education Project successfully applied for a grant to fund professional development programs for teachers in rural centers in two states. While the programs in each state differed in detail, they had the following common elements:

- focus on the teaching of literacy, involvement of a defined cluster of schools in a rural area;
- involvement of staff from a rural community college;
- release of teachers from classes to take part in a meaningful professional development activity;
- support from a coordinating agency with interests in rural education for schools and the community.

The program was initially offered at two sites.

In the planning stage, evaluators who had considerable empathy with the philosophy of the CEP were asked to undertake an evaluation of the program. A second reason for choosing these evaluators was that they had a strong conceptual knowledge of professional development. The clients were sure that the evaluators would provide plausible conclusions that could be used to refine the program. Following observations and interviews at the sites, a discussion paper was prepared by the evaluators. This was the basis of a series of meetings at which changes to the program for subsequent implementations were decided (Johnson & Owen 1995).

Ongoing cooperation over time

A way of increasing the use of evaluation findings is for evaluators and agencies to cooperate in partnership on several related studies over time. Huberman (1987) described the most effective partnerships in terms of 'sustained interactivity'. In this arrangement, the use of informal linkage mechanisms in addition to formal ones was simply activated when a particular study was required, and communication about the findings was set in motion. This effort relied on a lot of dissemination and utilization 'savviness', which Huberman maintains is probably the single most powerful influence on evaluation use.

When an individual study commenced, important communication strategies were as follows:

- interim feedback provided conceptual understandings of the progress of a study and tentative findings, and the opportunity for practitioners to understand the implications for local action. Through this there were chances for researchers to correct eventual misrepresentations;
- frequent, extensive and informal linkages between evaluators and users meant that exchanges were made with a minimum of defensiveness on either side; and
- commitment of both sides to consider, from an early stage, the implications of a study for action (Huberman & Cox 1990).

These observations show the strong interaction between personal relationships and use of evaluation findings. Other commentators have suggested that practitioners should become part of the evaluation team. This leads not only to the acquisition of inquiry skills, but also increases the likelihood that practitioners will act strategically in the implementation of the findings at the local level.

Example 11.3 Evaluation at Collingwood College

Over a period of ten years a university evaluation center undertook a series of evaluation studies at Collingwood College, a P–12 school in inner-city Melbourne. Prior to the first study, evaluation center staff and school administrators went to some lengths to identify how the two parties would operate. On the basis of the success of a first study, a series of additional studies has been commissioned. Despite changes in senior staff at the school and the evaluation center, cooperative arrangements have been maintained. Both parties have benefited from the relationship. The school has developed a reputation as a 'learning organization'. While at one time it was in danger of closing, it is now seen as a 'good school', responding to the needs of a changing community. In return, the school has allowed the evaluation center to use evaluation experiences at the school for teaching and research by its graduate students.

Interactive evaluation and organizational change

In practice, ongoing reporting to influence change has its challenges. While laying out findings to staff may merely involve setting up a meeting at which these can be presented, it is more difficult to get staff to focus on the implications of the findings for their collective practice.

Example 11.4 Saturn School

Preskill (1992) reports on a case study of an internal evaluation at Saturn School in Minnesota that adopted an innovatory program in which the roles of teachers, pupils and the parent community were redefined. Among other features, the curriculum of the school was developed from the information gathered from teachers and students. The curriculum was changed every ten weeks. Preskill was employed as a 'neutral force' evaluator to document the implementation of the curriculum and to provide systematic feedback to assist in its development. While her role as a documentor was appreciated, Preskill became frustrated with her influence on decision-making.

> As time went on into the second year . . . I became frustrated by my seeming inability to positively affect the school. I was sitting on so much data—information from all perspectives that seemed to be sealed within individuals or small groups of people. I increasingly felt ineffective in my ability to do what I had hoped—to provide ongoing information to the teachers and other staff about how things were going and to help them implement their mission more effectively. (p. 8)

On the basis of this experience, Preskill believes that organizations need to adjust their perspectives on organizational learning in order to use evaluation findings effectively. She notes that while individual teachers and others continually learnt from the evaluation and used the evaluator in many different ways, the organization as a whole was unable to develop a process whereby the staff could collaboratively reflect on the findings and apply them to the issues and problems associated with the innovation. Preskill analyzes this in terms of the need for organizations to develop structures within which evaluation can be used to restructure organizational norms, strategies and assumptions, known as 'double-loop' learning.

An implication for evaluators is that they need to be competent in facilitating group work and managing conflict. We have found from our practice that it is essential that the findings of the evaluation can provide a neutral force when there are existing and competing positions within an organization. In these situations, it is essential that all parties have absorbed the findings of the evaluation. Thus the evaluator must be prepared to give time to dissemination—in particular, to face-to-face dissemination. This often provides a means by which the organization can go forward on the basis of the input from the 'third party'.

Practitioner-led evaluation

Another issue is the extent to which practitioners should and do become involved in evaluation. In highly participatory site-based evaluations, practitioners could be involved in all phases: negotiating the key questions, collecting and analyzing evidence and reporting to colleagues.

For example, as part of a commitment to local control over schooling, evaluation could be used for the following reasons:

- The school council might want to revise and update the school policy so that it meets current needs.
- Students may feel that the curriculum and organization of the school are not adequately preparing them for adult life.
- One group of teachers may want to introduce a change that will impinge on other areas of the school.
- There is a change of policy (for example from the school district) necessitating a new look at the school's practices and priorities.

Whatever the object of the evaluation, it is clear that self-evaluation is action focused and orientated towards innovatory practice.

Anecdotal evidence suggests that schools respond favorably to these principles if they are given guidelines and support. The extent of commitment and quality of practice within school-level evaluation has surprised some evaluation theorists. For example, McLaughlin (in Alkin 1990) makes the following comment about school-level evaluation as practiced in Australia:

> [Practitioner-led evaluation], I think that's a fantastic way to go and in fact I have seen it work. But what seems to have gone along with it is, in addition to responsibility for evaluation, the authority to act on the results. That is not seen to be as an empty 'formal' kind of exercise. And I'm thinking particularly of schools I've seen in Australia, in which I was blown away with the really hard-nosed look they were taking at their own school. I thought, God, how did this happen? They

were asking tough questions. When I asked them about that, it turned out that they also had the power to make changes—they could make their schools better, based on the results. They worked with outside evaluators. They did a school-based review every two years. And it was really tough nosed.

While there has been enthusiastic system-level support for site-level evaluation in education, this has not always been matched in schools themselves, as teachers find that additional work burdens accrue. Wise school administrations have limited the number and scope of their formal evaluation work, concentrating on perhaps one major and a small number of minor evaluations a year and heeded advice to use outsiders in a supporting role.

Participant involvement

It is also possible for program participants to become involved in Interactive evaluation studies.

Example 11.5 Older persons as evaluators

The Adult Community and Further Education Board (ACFEB) provided support for the educational needs of persons over sixty years of age across eleven districts. Within each region, educational programs were provided through agencies such as neighborhood houses and community centers. An evaluation term was commissioned to answer the following questions:

- What is the existing pattern of provision of educational programs for older persons?
- What are the barriers to participation?
- What should the pattern of provision be in the future, say, for the next five to ten years?

A feature of the evaluation design was the involvement of older persons themselves, all of whom attended agencies that conducted the programs. They were involved in:

- door-to-door collection of information from program stakeholders;
- focus groups, acting as assistant moderators;

- entering evidence into databases;
- analyses of the findings;
- writing drafts of the reports; and
- organizing a conference where the findings were presented and discussed.

The leader of the evaluation team, Rosalind Hurworth, coordinated strategies to ensure rigor of the study. For example, she developed the interview schedule for the door-to-door information collection and trained the data collectors and focus group moderators. She identified participants who possessed data analytical skills, and coordinated the report writing. An unexpected outcome was that, for some time after the study ended, the city-based evaluation team became the 'place to visit' for country-based participants when they happened to be in town.

On reflection, the evaluators found the strategies used to be exciting but demanding, in that they:

- required more than the usual administrative work for the professionals involved;
- depended on the ability of the lead evaluator to rapidly build rapport; and
- demanded greater personal commitment from the evaluator than more conventional Interactive studies (Hurworth & Clemans 1996).

Organizationally integrated evaluation

An evaluator might perform a range of roles in an Interactive study. In addition to bringing a critical perspective, the external evaluator may be employed as a coordinator of the effort, for staff training and in areas where technical and methodological skills are needed.

In a project built around the provision of support groups designed to prevent or delay the use of drugs by young people, Dugan (1996) developed a five-stage model to evaluate these programs. The stages were:

- organizing for action;
- building the capacity for action;
- taking action;
- refining the action;
- institutionalizing the action.

Dugan undertook the following roles: facilitator, mentor, advocate, trainer, coach and 'expert', and documented the proportion of time devoted to these tasks at each stage. She spent 20 percent of her time in the organizing for action stage, and 40 percent in the 'building for capacity' and 'taking action' stages. Providing expertise grew from a small proportion in stage one (10 percent) to 50 percent in the 'refining the action' stage. While this example was developed within the Empowerment Approach, it could just as easily have been classed as Action Research. In fact, when Rowe and Jacobs (1996) undertook a similar study in a local evaluation of a Native American community, they regarded it as an Action Research study.

However, both Dugan, and Rowe and Jacobs, would subscribe to the following propositions:

- Evaluation is something that ordinary people can be involved in.
- Evaluation is guided by three tenets: it should be participatory, as systematic as possible, and at the same time, use simple methodologies.
- Evaluation should strive to address key issues, not prove hypotheses.
- Findings that have the potential to transfer benefits from one situation to another should be described in simple lessons-learned statements.
- People 'on the ground', not agencies or experts, are responsible for their own development (Dugan 1996).

There is, not surprisingly, an overlap in the methods used and the assumptions made about action across the Approaches in the Interactive Form.

CONCLUSION

One way of distinguishing between the Forms of evaluation is to identify the timing of an evaluation in relation to program planning and delivery. For example, a Proactive evaluation is undertaken before the related program is delivered, a Clarificative evaluation is located at the planning-into-action stage, while an Impact evaluation should focus on a mature program. The Interactive Form is more difficult to locate along this continuum, and in that sense is distinct from other Forms. At one time, Interactive Approaches were associated with program (and organizational) processes, which implied a focus on program delivery. However, it has been forcefully pointed out to us that Interactive studies can focus on outcomes. And, as can be seen from Example 11.5 above, an Interactive evaluation can use techniques that are consistent with needs assessment, which we have classified as a proactive technique in the Evaluation Forms (Chapter 3).

So timing may not distinguish Interactive evaluation from other Forms. Perhaps the clearest indicators are control of the evaluation process, location of the evaluation, and degree of participation in the evaluation process. Even then, there will be variations in each of these indicators depending on the Approach or Approaches adopted. However, a study heavily based on the Interactive Form would exhibit the following characteristics:

- it would be undertaken within an agency or organization; and
- control of the evaluation and use of findings are the responsibility of agency managers, providers and, in some instances, program beneficiaries.

REFERENCES

Alkin, M. C. (1990). *Debates on Evaluation.* Newbury Park, CA: Sage.

Brown, L. (1990). Self-evaluation for system management. Melbourne: Office of Schools Administration, Ministry of Education.

Cousins, J. B. and Earl, L. M. (1992). 'The Case for participatory evaluation'. *Educational Evaluation and Policy Analysis*, 14(4), 397–418.

Cousins, J. B. and Whitmore, E. (1998). Framing participatory evaluation. *New Directions for Evaluation,* 80 (Winter), 5–23.

Cuttance, P. (1994). *Quality Systems for the Performance Development Cycle of Schools.* Paper presented at the International Conference on School Effectiveness and Improvement (ICSEI), Melbourne, January 1994.

Dugan, M. A. (1996). Participatory and empowerment evaluation: Lessons learned in training and technical assistance. In D. M. Fetterman, S. J. Kaftarian and A. Wandersman (eds), *Empowerment Evaluation: Knowledge and Tools for Self Assessment and Accountability.* Thousand Oaks, CA: Sage.

Fetterman, D. M. (1994). Empowerment evaluation. *Evaluation Practice,* 15(1), 1–15.

Fetterman, D. M., Kaftarian, S. J. and Wandersman, A. (1996). *Empowerment Evaluation: Knowledge and Tools for Self-Assessment and Accountability.* Thousand Oaks, CA: Sage.

Fetterman, D. M. and Wandersman, A. E. (2004). *Empowerment Evaluation Principles in Practice.* New York: Guilford Publications.

Garvin, D. A. (1995). Building a learning organization. *Harvard Business Review,* 71(4), 78–91.

Havelock, R. G. (1971). *Planning for Innovation through Dissemination and Utilization of Knowledge.* Ann Arbor, MI: Center for Research on Utilization of Scientific Knowledge.

Huberman, M. (1987). Steps toward an integrated model of research utilization. *Knowledge, Creation, Diffusion, Utilization,* 8(4), 586–611.

Huberman, M. and Cox, P. (1990). Evaluation utilization: Building links between action and reflection. *Studies in Educational Evaluation*, 16(1), 157–179.

Hurworth, R. and Clemans, A. (1996). Assessing the educational needs of the older adult: An empowerment model of research. In V. Minichiello, N. Chappell, H. Kendig and A. Walker (eds), *Sociology of Aging: International Perspectives*. Fitzroy, Vic: International Sociological Association.

Johnson, N. J. and Owen, J. M. (1995). *The Rural Professional Education Program: An Evaluation*. Prepared for the Country Education Project (Inc): Melbourne, Vic.

Karlsson Vestman, O. (2004). *Evaluation as Learning: A Study of Social Worker Education in Leningrad County* (Vol. Research Report 2004:8A). Eskilstuna, Sweden: Centrum for Välfärdsforskning and Mälardalen Evaluation Academy.

Kemmis, S. (1985). *The Action Research Planner*. Geelong: Deakin University Press.

Lewin, K. (1946). Action research and minority problems. *Journal of Social Issues*, 2(4), 41–56.

Orton, J. (1992). 'Notes for a Graduate Course in Action Research'. Draft Paper. Melbourne: Faculty of Education, The University of Melbourne.

Owen, J. M. (2003). Evaluation culture: A definition and analysis of its development within organizations. *Evaluation Journal of Australasia*, 3(1), 43–47.

Patton, M. Q. (1996). A world larger than formative and summative. *Evaluation Practice*, 17(2), 131–44.

Preskill, H. (1992). Riding the Roller Coaster of Educational reform: The ups and downs of evaluation practice. Paper presented at the annual meeting of the American Evaluation Association; Seattle WA. November 1992.

Rowe, W. and Jacobs, N. (1996). 'Principles and practice of organizationally integrated evaluation'. Personal communication, August.

Sowell, T. (1996). *Knowledge and Decisions*. New York: Basic Books.

Stake, R. E. (1980). Program evaluation, particularly responsive evaluation. In W. B. Dockrell and D. Hamilton (eds), *Rethinking Evaluation Research*. London: Hodder & Stoughton.

Stockdill, S., H. Baizerman, M. and Compton, D. W. (2002). Towards a definition of the ECB process: A conversation with the literature. *New Directions for Evaluation*, 93, 7–24.

Torres, R. T. (2001). *Internal Evaluation and Organizational Development: Similarities, Differences and Opportunities for Learning*. Paper presented at the Annual Meeting of the American Evaluation Association, St Louis, MO.

Wadsworth, Y. (1997). *Everyday Evaluation on the Run*. Sydney: Allen & Unwin.

Monitoring Evaluation

12

The upsurge in importance of evaluation consistent with the Monitoring Form can be associated with two major trends in public policy. These are:

- increased accountability in government and non-profit sectors; and
- the emergence of performance-based management as the means for fulfilling these accountability requirements.

Monitoring evaluation can be regarded as a component of the current total quality management and quality assurance thrusts, made manifest in the United States through the *Government Performance and Results Act* (GPRA), enacted in 1993. Similar trends can be seen worldwide—for example, some member countries of the Organization for Economic Cooperation and Development (OECD) introduced performance-based management that required regular evaluation as long ago as 1987 (Mackay 2003).

These developments have wide-ranging implications for management, who now must be concerned with performance measurement—assembling evidence to show results—in addition to managing the planning and delivery of programs.

It is clear that there is a need for guidelines by which management can plan and implement evaluative schemes designed to monitor the performance of programs and organizations for accountability purposes. However, monitoring should also be designed to provide management with feedback that can be used to improve what is offered. Serving both accountability and improvement purposes provides a challenge for those evaluators who believe that performance-based management leads to more enlightened management and more effective delivery of services (Bernstein 1999).

Monitoring evaluation is associated with:

- checking that the delivery of articulated Program plans are on-track and that specified levels of outcomes specified are being achieved;

- developing management information systems (MIS) that can provide responsive, valid and useful information for assessing Program delivery and outcomes;
- providing evidence through which managers can report on the achievements to funding agencies and other stakeholders, including the public; and
- developing mechanisms by which Programs can be fine-tuned on the basis of the findings provided.

Features of this Form are included in Table 12.1.

KEY APPROACHES TO MONITORING EVALUATION

An analysis of existing patterns of Program management suggests three major Approaches within this Form of evaluation:

- component analysis;
- devolved performance assessment; and
- systems analysis.

Component analysis

In this Approach, senior management selects a component of the Program for systematic analysis and review, and assesses that component both in terms of its own objectives, and in terms of its contribution to the mission and overall goals of the Program.

In this Approach, the selection of the component for intensive study is made on the grounds of concern—for example, the component appears to be running poorly, or its outcomes are not as expected, or the component is a new or high-cost intervention that must be justified to a funding agency. The organization's internal evaluation capacity is directed to concentrate its energies on this component for a defined period.

Key assumptions underlying this approach are that senior management:

- has sufficient overview of the organization to be able to identify a component for attention;
- has the power to direct evaluation capacity to address the issue;
- is a major audience for the evaluation findings.

Devolved performance assessment

A second Approach is for senior management to encourage all components of a Program to have their performance assessed on a regular

Table 12.1 Summary of Monitoring evaluation

Dimension	Properties
Orientation	Assessing Program processes and outcomes, for fine-tuning and to account for Program resources
Typical issues	• Is the Program reaching the target population? • Is implementation meeting Program objectives and benchmarks? • How is implementation going between sites? • How is implementation now compared with a month ago? • How can we fine-tune this Program to make it more efficient? • How can we fine-tune this Program to make it more effective? • Is there a Program site which needs attention to ensure more effective delivery?
State of program	Settled; Program plan is in place
Major focus	Delivery and outcomes
Timing (vis-à-vis Program delivery)	During delivery
Key Approaches	• Component analysis • Devolved performance assessment • Systems analysis
Assembly of evidence	Relies on the meaningful use of valid performance measures to produce performance information. In some cases this will be in the form of quantitative indicators. Systems approach relies on the availability of a management information system (MIS) which includes the capacity to develop the indicators.

basis. Senior management receives these reports and, using appropriate criteria, makes judgments on the contribution of each component to the mission and overall goals of the organization. Decisions about changes to one or more components are made in the light of these judgments.

In this approach, senior management is expected to provide guidelines and resources for undertaking component evaluations, and principles for judging the relative contributions of each component, should this be necessary. In this approach, field staff may be expected to implement the evaluation of the component in which they are located, perhaps with assistance from a central evaluation unit.

Systems analysis

The third Approach applies to a Program that is centrally specified and disseminated for implementation to a large number of sites. The Program specification includes a set of important goals. Guidelines are provided for field staff to aid implementation. Field staff have little or no say in Program specification or implementation plans.

An evaluation scenario consistent with this design involves:

- a set of important outcomes to be defined and made operational;
- using a centralized evaluation capacity to compare directly the performance of sites using the same operational criteria; and
- relating differences in attainment of the outcomes to differences in Program delivery across sites. In this way, statements about the relative effectiveness of each site can be made.

Key evaluation questions are:

- Is the Program reaching the target population?
- Is it being implemented in the ways specified?
- Is it effective?
- How much does it cost?
- What are the costs relative to its effectiveness?

This systems Approach to evaluation developed in the United States in the mid- to late-1960s (Rossi & Freeman 1989). While a central management information system (MIS) would be useful for all three Approaches, it is essential for systems analysis, where it provides the basis for creating relevant indications of the relative effectiveness and efficiency of a Program at different sites. While the creation of a large-scale MIS that is easy to manage and responsive seems to be a feasible proposition, there are few case examples which illustrate the advantages of such a system for Program management. This and associated issues are discussed in the next section.

MONITORING EVALUATION: TRENDS AND CASE EXAMPLES

As indicated in the introduction to this chapter, two major trends related to monitoring evaluation are: the emergence of accountability, and developments in performance management. These are discussed, in turn, below.

Accountability

Monitoring evaluation is often undertaken for accountability purposes. This section focuses on meanings of accountability and the use of evaluation to justify spending on interventions at organizational and system levels. There is no doubt that accountability concerns are paramount in the private sector. The collapse of large corporations in the United States and elsewhere has led to an erosion of confidence in the quality of financial accounting standards and the behavior of senior executives. The very fabric of economic life in Western societies has been called into question. Governments have introduced measures designed to restore confidence in the stock market, and to punish company directors and others who have attempted to defraud their shareholders.

Concern for accountability is also apparent in the public sector. The public wants to be satisfied that spending on public sector programs and institutions is both effective and efficient (Gilbert 1998). Accountability is a catchcry in today's public sector politics.

Associated with the increased emphasis on accountability is a connection with the use of performance information to show that programs are meeting targets and providing value for money (Ryan 2002). The need for such information is particularly evident in the United States following the passage of the GPRA, which requires federal public authorities to specify and report on the achievement or otherwise of stated program objectives (Gordon & Heinrech 2004).

However, there is a danger that strident calls for accountability can lead to systemic arrangements which can have deleterious effects on the quality of programs and the clients of these programs, resulting in outcomes which are the opposite to those they are designed to achieve (Earl & Lafleur 1997).

Meanings of accountability

What is meant by accountability? Related to the education sector, accountability has been described as:

> the responsibility for the justification of expenditures, decisions, or results of one's own efforts. Program managers and teachers should be, it is often said, accountable for their salaries and expenditures and time, or accountable for pupils' achievement, or both (Scriven 1991, p. 46).

In terms of programmatic interventions accountability represents an obligation on the part of managers to report on the exercise of their responsibilities, the expenditure of funds and the implementation of mandated activities.

Accountability thus seems to involve a transaction along the lines of 'if we give you the resources, we expect you to show us what you have achieved with them'. For an individual professional practitioner the resources are in form of a salary; for a programmatic intervention, the resources are those that fund that intervention. The conventional accountability process transaction is based around the flow of funds in one direction and the flow of related information in the other.

How does *accountability* differ from *responsibility*? We think that they are similar, with the exception that accountability implies greater consequences for the personnel involved. Accountability includes sanctions whereas responsibility does not. Sanctions can come in many forms and are worn by those responsible for the intervention being delivered. The result of an accountability transaction might be a reprimand for the program director, a note on an employment file, a promotion denied, or even the loss of job.

We recall a senior public servant responsible for radical changes in a school system in the early 1990s remarking that if the findings of a review showed that a school was 'failing', the school could be closed or a principal could be dismissed. This raises the issue of attribution and fairness. It seems that one can only be accountable for actions over which one has direct control. However, we are aware that the traditional Westminster system of government assumes that a Minister is responsible for his or her department, and that, if a major impropriety occurs, the Minister traditionally takes the blame for this indiscretion and offers to resign. This is despite the fact that the Minister cannot possibly exert control over all the events that are handled by the department, or over the decisions of public servants at all levels within the bureaucracy.

Concerns about consequences are a key concern for senior staff responsible for implementing government policy. While they have lived with accountability on a day-to-day basis in the past, these concerns seem to be heightened when performance information is available about interventions for which they have responsibility.

Roles for evaluation in accountability

As we have indicated in Chapter 9, a new age of evidence-based decision-making has emerged which has implications for accountability systems. Observers suggest that, while professional judgment and opinion were once regarded as sufficient, they no longer have widespread acceptance as a means of confirming the effectiveness of programs (Reed & Brown 2001).

This seems an appropriate place to summarize the 'state of play' about accountability and evaluation practice. In doing so, we rely heavily on recent North American evaluation research and ask readers to extrapolate these findings to their own contexts.

Accountability systems that have emerged over the last decade are characterized by the following:

- increased community interest in what has been achieved for the expenditure of funds on social programs (Segerholm 2003), and more attention to the demands of consumers in the planning of public programs;
- devolution of authority from the center to departments and agencies, with the proviso that they will report on program effectiveness;
- monitoring evaluation being increasingly integrated into accountability arrangements at whole-of-government and departmental levels;
- differing accountability imperatives emerging, dependent on the position of audiences in the program provision hierarchy. For example, (1) fiscal and overall performance reporting 'up' from government departments to centralized fiscal agencies responsible for budget allocations, compared with (2) emphasis on program performance within a department from program manager to the senior executive (Ryan 2002);
- evidence collected by organizations in management information systems (MIS) unable to meet the accountability needs of all stakeholder groups;
- lack of evaluation expertise at department and agency level, particularly in not-for-profit agencies, which impacts on the quality of evidence collected and disseminated (Poole et al. 2000), and the need to divert program development resources to evaluation (Ryan et al. 1996);
- evaluation being incorrectly equated with the development and application of performance indicators and the inability of indicators to adequately tap the range of outcomes of a given intervention (Schalock & Bonham 2003);
- widespread concern that accountability information which is reported up a hierarchy is not being used for decision-making at the next level of that hierarchy (Leighton 2003);

- inability of outcome-focused frameworks to provide practitioners with information that will lead to improvements in program provision, despite this being a key rationale for governments embracing accountability systems (Ryan 2002); and
- a need for champions of accountability to embrace a wider view of 'what counts' as evidence for the purposes of public responsibility (Wholey et al. 1994; Feller 2002).

Performance management

In evaluative terms, there are strong links between accountability and performance management, which can be thought of as the routine measurement, analysis and reporting of program performance. This involves managers in the use of 'performance information in systems for managing their agencies and programs, in accountability to key stakeholders and to the public to demonstrate effective and improved performance, and to support resource allocation and other policy decision-making' (Wholey 1999).

Example 12.2 Encouraging the use of performance measures

A survey of federal government agencies conducted by the US General Accounting Office found that the most difficult challenges in developing performance measures were: (a) getting beyond outputs to develop outcome measures; and (b) specifying quantifiable performance indicators. Strategies which had been used to develop outcome measures included:

- developing a measurement model that encompassed state and local activity to identify outcome measures for federal programs;
- encouraging program managers to develop different funding scenarios;
- conceptualizing the outcomes of daily activities;
- planning and implementing customer satisfaction and developing multiple measures of satisfaction;
- using qualitative measures of outcomes; and
- involving stakeholders (GAO 1997).

While the impact of performance management has been most pervasive in the United States, it is now in widespread use in countries in the

Organization for Economic Cooperation and Development (OECD) and the developing world. An important finding across these countries is that when a government signals its intentions to focus on program results, rather than inputs, the overall performance of the program improves.

While the US-based research paints a generally negative picture of the impact of performance management regimes, there are instances where such a regime has had some positive outcomes. An example is a Program known as 'Schools of the Future', located in Australia. To bring to the fore some of the positive trends in the practice of performance management, we discuss this case in detail below.

Schools of the Future required all government schools (in the State of Victoria) to:

- develop a strategic planning document, known as a 'school charter'. This was a plan for the work of the school for the next three years, to identify its long-term goals and implementation strategies, as well as how it would implement government priorities, such as a state-wide focus on literacy;
- provide summaries of achievements of these plans, based heavily on quantitative indicator evidence. This required that findings be sent from all schools to the Department of Education (DOE) to meet accountability requirements set by the government. This information was forwarded as annual reports that were also available to the school community, and as triennial reports, which followed a major review of the information that had been assembled, over a three year period. The findings enabled the DOE to compare the performance of all government schools in the state.

During this period, each school was also asked to monitor its progress towards the achievement of school charter goals. This was achieved by the application of monitoring tools developed by the DOE, such as parent satisfaction scales, and the interrogation of information provided to it by the DOE—for example, its performance on statewide tests in the areas of numeracy and literacy.

This evaluation and reporting regime was originally designed for accountability purposes, but it was later modified to include the use of the information to assist schools in making decisions about improvements to their strategic plans.

A review of the impact of Schools of the Future policy found the following:

- Implementation involved significant additional work by staff, especially by the principal.
- Schools were not accustomed and generally did not have the evaluation skills to collect and analyze the data that had to be collected.

- Many of the indicators employed related to administrative rather than educational aspects of the work of the schools.
- Changes and additions to the roles of school leaders during this time represented an enormous challenge to principals and other staff (Owen 2003).

These findings are consistent with the research literature on flaws associated with introduction of performance management systems in government and not-for-profit agencies. However, the fact that the DOE finally encouraged the use of performance information for improvement purposes led to a change in opinions about the collection of use of this information at school level. This was achieved through the persistence and assistance of sympathetic external reviewers drawn from universities and other institutions. We now find, a decade after the introduction of Schools of the Future, that principals are more likely to use performance information as a means of leading staff discussions on school outcomes and procedures. The availability of 'independent' evidence has become more persuasive than staff opinion and speculation about how the school is performing. Over time, there has also been a turnaround in staff attitudes towards the role of such evidence as one input into organizational decision-making.

Moving from this example to the research literature on performance management and the roles of monitoring, several points can be made:

1 There is no doubt that performance management is now part of the mainstream of evaluation practice. Well-known evaluators such as Joseph Wholey, Kathryn Newcomer and Arnold Love have dedicated a substantial part of their careers to advancing practice and theory related to this aspect of the Monitoring Form.
2 While some theorists do not regard monitoring and performance measurement as a Form of evaluation, many program managers disagree with this conceptual distinction. These managers would subscribe to the view that:

   Performance management involves more than simply recording measures of programmatic performance and reporting them upwards in agencies, to oversight bodies and stakeholders of public programs. Several steps are needed to develop and collect performance measures that can be useful to management in decision-making:

   - program stakeholders must come to some reasonable agreement on strategic and performance objectives and the strategies for achieving them;
   - indicators must be defined for program components that capture program outputs or outcomes;

- data sources must be developed with systematic methods, often in multiple jurisdictions (for example, states, grant-funded projects, etc.);
- data must be aggregated and reported in data-friendly formats;
- the data must be used by program managers and decision-makers to assess and improve results; and
- data quality must be addressed at every step of the journey from original collection to final reporting (Scheirer & Newcomer 2001).

3 One of the major criticisms leveled at performance measurement is the separation of cause and effect. There are several explanations for this:

- Outcomes information is the major form of evidence generally required by high-level decision-makers such as legislative committees and funding sources. These bodies are more concerned with the level of performance an intervention attains relative to the set target, than with how that performance was achieved.
- Separation of cause and effect suits some managers. While outcomes data collected by rigorous means is welcome, they believe that their own knowledge and insights are sufficient for them to make changes to their organization and the programs they oversee.
- Undertaking a rigorous analysis of causes may not be possible due to limitation of time, or programmatic causes may be too complex—for example, the level at which the data is collected, such as aggregation at the mega program level, or where more than one Program is likely to have contributed to a given outcome. Methodologies that address contribution rather than attribution are still in early stages of development.

4 Nevertheless, the use of program logic based on the intentions of a program can be of benefit in setting up a performance measurement system. Logic models can be based on the generic model shown in Figure 12.1.

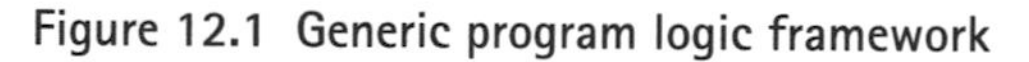
Figure 12.1 Generic program logic framework

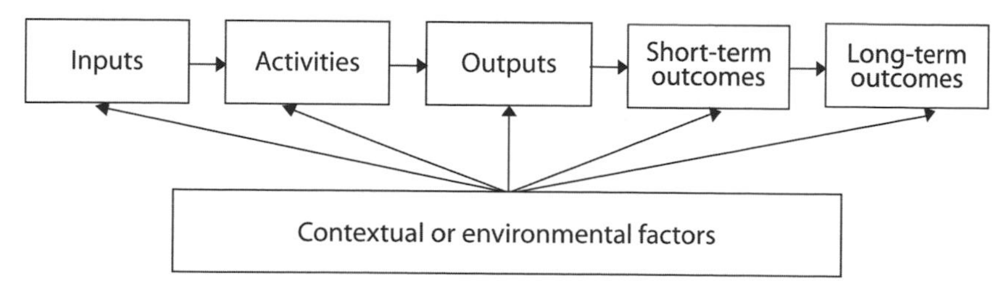

A program logic framework encourages managers to identify where a given variable of interest is located—for example, whether it is best classified as an activity or an outcome. Decisions about which variables should be measured can also be clarified from the logic model. It is also possible to set up evaluation studies that explore a causal link by identifying variables of interest in the logic. In fact, examples of studies of this nature are beginning to appear in the literature (Scheirer 2000).

The efficacy of performance management in contributing to effective public sector program delivery was the subject of a major debate involving Perrin (1998), Bernstein (1999) and Winston (1999). Directions for improved performance management practice that arose from this debate are summarized below:

1 *Change the focus of accountability*
This involves transferring accountability requirements from meeting targets to becoming responsible for implementing outcome-focused evaluation procedures. This requires managers to show that they are concerned with the use of performance information to make their programs more effective and efficient. Under such a scheme, managers would no longer be accountable for meeting program targets over which they did not have total control, but would be accountable for encouraging a commitment to evidence-based practice and improvement in their organization.

2 *Emphasize performance information rather than performance indicators or measures*
An indicator or measure can be thought of as a construct or variable which is amenable to measurement. Usually indicators are presented in quantitative format. While some indicator data may summarize simple variables in the form of counts or ratios, others may report more complex information such as an aggregated score on an attitude scale that is composed of several items.

Performance indicators or measures can be considered as the data collection aspect of data management. The analysis and interpretation of these measures leads to performance information about a given intervention.

Evaluators need to understand this distinction and to recognize that analysis and interpretation of indicator data is essential for the production of valid and meaningful findings. According to Perrin (1999), emphasizing performance information rather than performance measures is a way forward in determining the achievement of public programs.

3 *Use program logic to prioritize evaluation needs*
This was discussed above.

4 *Keep in mind the truth and utility trade-off*
Perrin (1999) distinguishes between 'bad data' and 'dirty data'. Bad data are irrelevant, untrustworthy or misleading—for example, the results of a survey with a low response rate purporting to provide accurate population norms. Dirty data is approximate rather than exact, and not definitive. However, such data can provide the minimum evidence needed to provide the minimum amount of extra confidence about a pending decision. As such it might be used in conjunction with an existing and more comprehensive body of information, and, tip the balance between alternative actions.
5 *Accept the limitations of measurement*
Perrin appeals to the views of gurus of management theory, who advance a view that assessment of the success of many government activities requires 'soft judgment', which cannot be provided by hard evidence.
6 *Consider alternative methods for judging success*
One example is a performance story (Dart & Mayne 2005). A performance story is a summary of the performance of a program that describes the causal links that show how achievement came about. Performance stories have been deployed in Canada and elsewhere. They are developed around a tentative program logic for the program. In addition to use for accountability purposes, performance stories discuss what was learned and so can provide directions for program improvement.

CONCLUSION

Developments related to the Monitoring Form of evaluation have been far-reaching and extensive during the past decade. In the early 1990s, the major concerns related to what constituted the characteristics of a performance indicator (Winston 1991). There was always concern about the need to use a range of indicators, and program evaluators were concerned with trade-offs between indicators which measured appropriateness, efficiency and effectiveness.

The accountability in government movement has forced us to lift our eyes to see the location of the Monitoring Form in terms of, first of all, within a more general evaluation framework, and also in terms of the broader political and economic developments of recent times.

REFERENCES

Bernstein, D. J. (1999). Comments on Perrin's 'Effective use and misuse of performance measurement'. *American Journal of Evaluation*, 20(1), 85–93.

Dart, J. and Mayne, J. (2005). Performance story. In S. Matheson (ed.), *Encyclopedia of Evaluation* (pp. 306–308). Thousand Oaks, CA: Sage.

Earl, L. and Lafleur, C. E. (1997). Forging a link between accountability and improvement in schools. *Orbit*, 28(3), 3–52.

Feller, I. (2002). Performance measurement redux. *American Journal of Evaluation*, 23(4), 435–452.

General Accounting Office (1997). *Managing for results: Analytical challenges in measuring performance*. GAO/HEH/GGD–97–138. Washington, DC: GAO.

Gilbert, A. D. (1998). *Ensuring Accountability*. Melbourne: The University of Melbourne.

Gordon, R. A. and Heinrech, C. J. (2004). Modeling trajectories in social program outcomes for performance accountability. *American Journal of Evaluation*, 25(2), 161–189.

Leighton, B. (2003). *Evaluation and Accountability*. Paper presented at the Annual Meeting of the American Evaluation Association, November 2003, Reno, NV.

Mackay, K. (2003). Two generations of performance evaluation and management systems in Australia. *Canberra Bulletin of Public Administration*, (110), 9–19.

Owen, J. M. (2003). Evaluating educational programs and projects in Australia. In T. Kellaghan and D. L. Stufflebeam (eds), *International Handbook of Educational Evaluation* (pp. 751–768). Dordrecht: Kluwer Academic Publishers.

Perrin, B. (1998). Effective use and misuse of performance measurement. *American Journal of Evaluation*, 19(3), 367–379.

Perrin, B. (1999). Performance measurement: Does the reality match the rhetoric? A rejoinder to Bernstein and Perrin. *American Journal of Evaluation*, 20(1), 101–111.

Poole, D. L., Carnahan, S., Chepnick, N. G. and Tubiak, C. (2000). Evaluating performance measurement systems in non-profit agencies. *American Journal of Evaluation*, 21(1), 15–26.

Reed, C. S. and Brown, R. E. (2001). Outcome–asset impact model: Linking outcomes and assets. *Evaluation and Program Planning*, 95(3), 287–295.

Rossi, P. H. and Freeman, H. E. (1989). *Evaluation: A Systematic Approach*, 4th ed. Newbury Park, CA: Sage.

Ryan, K. (2002). Shaping educational accountability systems. *American Journal of Evaluation*, 23(4), 453–468.

Ryan, K., Geissier, B. and Knell, S. (1996). Progress and accountability in family literacy. *Evaluation and Program Planning*, 23(2), 263–272.

Schalock, R. L. and Bonham, G. S. (2003). Measuring outcomes and managing for results. *Evaluation and Program Planning*, 26(2), 229–235.
Scheirer, M. A. (2000). Getting more bang for your performance measure buck. *American Journal of Evaluation*, 21(2), 139–149.
Scheirer, M. A. and Newcomer, K. E. (2001). Opportunities for program evaluators to facilitate performance-based management. *Evaluation and Program Planning*, 24, 63–71.
Scriven, M. (1991). *Evaluation Thesaurus,* 4th ed. Newbury Park, CA: Sage.
Segerholm, C. (2003). Researching evaluation in national (state) politics and administration: A critical approach. *American Journal of Evaluation*, 24(3), 353–372.
Wholey, J. S. (1999). Performance-based measurement: Responding to the challenge. *Public Productivity and Management Review*, 2(3), 288–307.
Wholey, J. S., Hatry, H. P. and Newcomer, K. E. (1994). *Handbook of Practical Program Evaluation*. San Francisco: Jossey-Bass.
Winston, J. A. (1991). *Linking Evaluation and Performance Management.* Paper presented at the Annual Conference of the Australasian Evaluation Society, Adelaide, SA.
Winston, J. A. (1999). Performance indicators—promises unmet: A response to Perrin. *American Journal of Evaluation*, 20(1), 95–99.

13 Impact Evaluation

Impact evaluation has a strong summative emphasis in that it provides findings from which a judgment of the worth of a program can be made. Impact evaluations are retrospective in that they occur at a logical point in time of program delivery to help us to take stock of that program. Ideally, Impact evaluations are undertaken on programs that are in a mature or settled stage and have had sufficient time to have an effect.

Impact evaluation rests partly on a not-unreasonable assumption that citizens at large should know whether programs funded by government, or in which they have an interest, are making a difference. Stakeholders expect that programs, where possible, meet their intended goals and do not lead to negative side-effects. Parents at a local school are interested in whether the literacy approach taken by that school is meeting the needs of their children. Likewise, those in management positions need to know whether the strategies they have selected to solve a given problem are being used and whether they work.

Accountability and Impact evaluation are related. As indicated in Chapter 12, a key element of the accountability thrust is that the public has a right to expect that funds spent in the public arena have been translated into effective social or educational interventions. For example, have the millions of dollars spent on making cities safer places led to a decrease in inner-city crime?

In addition to accountability, Impact evaluation can be used in making decisions about the future of the program under review. Ideally, programs should be trialed before they are distributed more widely. This was the original rationale for evaluation during the 1960s and 1970s, and underlies the work of influential practitioners such as Donald Campbell.

Consider the case of a new road safety program being implemented as a trial in one location. The program is sponsored by a government department, which is considering the expansion of the program to other locations. An Impact evaluation of the trial program is undertaken to test its effectiveness. In this case it would be important for the evaluation to focus on both the outcome and implementation elements of the program.

It is not uncommon for commissioners of an evaluation to ask for an Impact evaluation on an immature program. Those responsible for the evaluation need to educate commissioners and clients that as a result of doing so, they (the commissioners) may prematurely judge and terminate a program that, with some improvements, might become effective.

Impact evaluation is concerned with:

- determining the range and extent of outcomes of a program;
- determining whether a program has been implemented as planned and how implementation has affected outcomes;
- providing evidence to funders, senior managers and politicians about the extent to which resources allocated to a program have been spent wisely; and
- informing decisions about replication or extension of a program.

Key aspects of the Impact evaluation Form are summarized in Table 13.1.

While some evaluators use the term 'impact' only to denote long-term cumulative effects of programs over time (Rugg et al. 2004), we will use 'impact' to mean both immediate and longer term effects, both intended and unintended. Usually, but not always, effects of programs are in terms of changes to program participants.

Outcomes are a major concern of Impact evaluation. What do we mean by an outcome? An outcome is the effect of program activities on target audiences or populations, such as change in knowledge, attitudes, beliefs, skills, access to services, policies and environmental conditions (Rugg et al. 2004, p. 10).

For a particular program, there may be various levels of outcomes, with one level of outcome leading to a 'higher' or longer term outcome (see Chapter 10 for a discussion of outcome hierarchies). Examples of outcomes include: increased knowledge about nutrition, changes in literacy levels, getting a job, having higher self-dependence. An example of a hierarchy of outcomes for a youth mentoring program could be: (a) attending school more regularly; (b) improved reading skills; (c) getting higher grades; (d) getting a job.

By comparison, *outputs* are products of the program's activities, such as the number of meals provided, classes taught, participants served, or materials distributed. An output can be thought of as a simple indicator of the influence of a program.

While program effects are of direct interest to stakeholders of the program under review, they can also be a source of information for

Table 13.1 Summary of Impact evaluation

Dimension	Properties
Orientation	Establishment of program worth Justification of decisions to mount the program Accountability to funders and other stakeholders
Typical issues	• Has the program been implemented as planned? • Have the stated goals of the program been achieved? • Have the needs of those served by the program been met? • What are the unintended outcomes? • Does the implementation strategy lead to intended outcomes? • How do differences in implementation affect program outcomes? • What are the benefits of the program given the costs?
State of program	Settled
Major focus	Focus on delivery and/or outcomes. Most comprehensive studies combine both delivery and outcomes known as process–outcome studies
Timing (vis-à-vis program delivery)	Nominally 'after' the program has completed at least one cycle with program beneficiaries. In practice, impact studies could be undertaken at any time after program is 'settled'.
Key Approaches	• Objectives-based • Needs-based • Goal-free • Process-outcome studies • Realistic evaluation • Performance audit
Assembly of evidence	Traditionally required use of preordinate research designs, where possible the use of treatment and control groups, and the use of tests and other quantitative data. Studies of implementation generally require observational data. Determining all the outcomes requires use of more exploratory methods and the use of qualitative evidence.

the wider community of scholars and policy-makers. Probably more than any other evaluation Form, Impact evaluation findings related to a given program may contribute to the 'funded knowledge' about a phenomenon of which the given program is typical. Most evaluators would agree that, individually, or by aggregating findings across similar programs, it is possible to arrive at generalizations about the phenomenon.

Thus, evaluation findings can contribute to the social science knowledge base. Given that most Impact evaluations are retrospective, their direct influence on the program being examined is obviously limited unless it is replicated. But the fact that the findings might be used more broadly provides those responsible for impact studies with an incentive to carry them out with rigor. For example, individual evaluation studies of training programs have shown the importance of transfer to the workplace of participants and the need for follow-up coaching. Meta-analyses of these studies have confirmed these findings across a range of contexts. These findings have implications for the policy on training and its implementation for the future (Guskey 1994).

KEY APPROACHES TO IMPACT EVALUATION

Impact evaluations are concerned with establishing what works and why. The Approaches within Impact evaluation represent the closest manifestation in the real world to the logic of evaluation that was discussed in Chapter 1. To be able to back up claims that a program is having an impact, we must translate the logic of evaluation principles into action. This involves selection of key variables, setting standards and accessing evidence from which we can determine the success or otherwise of the intervention. Impact evaluation provided the genesis of evaluation practice—in fact, for some time it was seen as the only Form of evaluation. While thinking about evaluation has progressed from this position, Impact evaluation is the evaluation Form which is most practiced. Thus it is important for evaluators to have a thorough grasp of the essentials of the Form. As can be seen from Table 13.1, six Approaches to Impact evaluation are included within the Form. These are:

- objectives-based;
- needs-based;
- goal-free;
- process–outcome studies;
- realistic evaluation; and
- performance audit.

These will now be discussed in turn.

Objectives-based

This Approach determines whether the stated goals or objectives of a program have been achieved. Tyler (1950), the father figure of evaluation, was the chief proponent of evaluation based on goal achievement. In this Approach, the goals of a program are taken as a given, and decisions about the success of the program are based on the extent to which goals are achieved, according to some standard or level of achievement. In some cases, these objectives are expressed in terms of gains in attainment of program participants.

This Approach is now employed as a tool of management in both the public and private sectors. Management by objectives is applied to the performance of organizations, to organizational units (Big P programs), and to individuals. In the latter situation, we move into the realms of assessment or appraisal rather than program evaluation. The development of fair and valid procedures for assessing the performance of individuals is a contentious area, because the results of performance appraisal have direct consequences for them. Staff can be demoted or promoted and salary bonuses are tied to the results of individual performance appraisals.

The translation of program goals or objectives into valid measures of outcomes involves a set of methodological decisions. It may be possible to use previously developed instrument(s), but the evaluator must be satisfied that the instrument has face validity and that the intended audience for the evaluation will find it a credible measure of the objective(s). There is a temptation to use 'off-the-shelf' instruments, even though they do not fully meet this validity test. Sometimes evaluators must develop instruments, so skill in developing tests and other outcome measures is called for. The main tasks in setting up an objectives-based evaluation are as follows:

- Determine whether a key issue for stakeholders is to check on the attainment of program outcomes. Bear in mind that the program should be 'settled' for an outcomes study to be credible (see Table 13.1).
- Determine the 'real' objectives or goals of the program. Possible sources of information about program goals include:
  - policy documents;
  - program statements;
  - interviews with program providers;
  - a combination of more than one of the above.
- Decide on the most appropriate ways to determine whether the program has led to the attainment of the goals—for example, with relation to the design of the data management, whether a 'control

group' is available, whether it is possible to use a 'before and after' design, and when one can collect outcome data.
- Select appropriate measuring instruments, or develop new ones. Considerations include consistency between the outcome variables and program goals, the style and content of instruments, and the items to be used. If the instrument has been developed for the purpose, it is preferable that it be subject to a trial.
- Identify the sources of evidence.
- Collect and analyze the evidence.
- Draw conclusions, in some cases make judgments based on explicit or implicit levels of attainment for the outcome variables, make recommendations.
- Report the findings.

Needs-based

An alternative to an objectives-based approach is to determine worth on the basis of whether a program meets an identifiable need. Thus, it is important that the nature and extent of need be established as the basis of structuring an Impact evaluation when this Approach is adopted. Needs-based evaluation was first suggested by Scriven (1972), in response to perceived limitations of the Objectives-based Approach. His argument hinged on the view that program objectives did not necessarily reflect the needs of the program participants.

Thus, while an objectives-based Approach is based on the internal consistency of a program, a needs-based Approach adopts an external point of reference for judging program worth. You will appreciate that, if program goals do reflect needs, then the objectives-based and needs-based findings should be similar. Most program developers attempt to reflect the needs of participants in their program design, but there are always programs that are developed without reference to the needs of participants. In fact, if a needs assessment is not undertaken, this leaves well-intentioned program developers reliant on other sources of information for their planning. This was discussed in Chapter 9. Of course, there are also instances where programs are developed without reference to participant needs—for example, if a program is 'thrown together' in order to spend unallocated resources at the end of a financial year.

Goal-free

The Goal-free Approach was also a reaction to a slavish acceptance of the Objectives-based Approach. In goal-free evaluation, the evaluator deliberately ignores the stated or intended goals of the program. The purpose is to examine all program effects, rather than limiting the investigation to outcomes which reflect program objectives. Practically, the notion of deliberately ignoring the intentions of a programmatic intervention borders on the bizarre. Commissioners and clients are almost always interested in whether program objectives have been met, and the evaluator would need to go to extremes to ignore information about how the program is meant to operate. So in practice, goal-free evaluations are rare. However, the notion of Goal-free has led to one important aspect of practice—examining unintended as well as intended outcomes. In almost every intervention there are outcomes that could not have been anticipated in advance of program provision. In some cases, they can be as important as the intended outcomes. For example, a well-known physics curriculum met its stated goals of increasing deeper understanding of physics principles among senior high school students. However, as a result of the pressure placed on students by the teaching methods used, their enjoyment of physics declined over the instruction period. This was a major unintended outcome. There was evidence that students were 'turned off' physics as a result of the curriculum, and this affected their subsequent decision to study the subject at college level.

Process-outcome studies

As we have seen, Impact evaluations examine mature programs to determine outcomes. It is often necessary to check on the extent of program implementation in order to explain the pattern of outcomes. Thus an examination of program implementation can be an integral part of an Impact evaluation.

Implementation is also an important phenomenon in its own right, for the very reason that it is an integral part of a program intervention. The importance of implementation emerged in the 1960s and 1970s, when large-scale centrally funded Programs were seen as the core of improvements in society. Examples include the design of national-level school curricula, the development and diffusion of agricultural innovations such as new strains of grain crops, and social-biotechnological initiatives such as birth control programs.

Many of these change proposals were based on a Research Development and Diffusion (RD&D) model of change. RD&D relies on centrally researched and developed solutions to problems that are then disseminated to field users. The RD&D paradigm reflected an engineering perspective towards change that had been successfully used in the development and use of products by industry, particularly within Western economies during the twentieth century.

Many of the educational reforms were based on variations of RD&D. It was assumed that, if the developers 'got it right', improvements in the field would automatically follow. All that was required was for practitioners to translate the program plan into action by following specified guidelines.

Early research on the impact of these programs concentrated on measuring outcomes. For many innovations, the findings were not impressive. For example, student learning gains, compared with more traditional teaching approaches, were small or non-existent. It was concluded that the innovative curricula were having minimal impact. They appeared to have been a waste of time and money.

However, some evaluators began to examine the implementation of these programs. Rather than assume that the new curricula *were* implemented in ways that were consistent with the intentions of program developers, evaluators began to look at what was actually happening in classrooms. When observations of programs in action were made, wide variations in the degree to which teachers actually implemented them were noted. Analyses showed that there was a strong correlation between student learning outcomes and degree of program implementation. This made an enormous difference to the conclusions about the effects of educational RD&D; the large-scale educational projects were making a difference when they *were* indeed implemented.

Studies of this kind are called process–outcome studies. The outcomes can be thought of as the 'dependent' variables and the implementation or process characteristics as the 'independent' variables.

A standard procedure in these studies is to administer tests that measure outcomes, as outlined earlier in this chapter. It is then necessary to determine the degree to which implementation action is consistent with the intentions of the program plan. While observation is the most frequently used method of data collection, there are examples of multiple measures of implementation, such as records, self-reports and interviews. Directions for the construction of schedules and for the ensuing collection of information are found in Morris and Fitzgibbon (1978).

Implementation as the dependent variable

There are some evaluative situations where outcome measures are not required. In these cases, implementation of a program becomes the end point of the study design.

A logical approach to measuring implementation is to derive a series of implementation characteristics from a program plan. This assumes that the plan is sufficiently well specified to include details of the expected program activities; this is known as a *fidelity approach* to measuring implementation.

Hall and his colleagues (Hall & Loucks 1979) designed a conceptual scheme for determining program implementation that acknowledged the importance of time as a variable. They found that staff responsible for the use of an innovative program move through stages of understanding and action that determine the state of implementation of the program. The stages are: non-use, orientation, preparation, mechanical use, routine, refinement, integration and renewal.

In a conceptual sense, fidelity-based evaluation concentrates on mechanical and routine use to the exclusion of other implementation effects. The evaluator develops measures of the essential features of the program in action. This is easier if the program has a well-defined simple logic—for example, programs that emphasize skills training.

Adaptation

There is evidence to show that a centrally developed intervention undergoes changes when implemented at the local level (Spillane et al. 2002). Most programs, and those who are implementing them, undergo a process of mutual adaptation during implementation. That is, the implementer alters her actions towards those specified by the program, but may not implement the program faithfully. The nature of the adaptation depends on local conditions and on the degree of support given by developers for the change. Program activities take shape slowly as providers react to the realities of the context with its emerging complexities.

This has implications for assessing the extent of implementation. To understand how and why programs are implemented differently in different locations, there is an argument for implementation evaluation to document variations in use, and the factors that lead to patterns of use at each location or site. Evaluation methods thus need to be more flexible than those used in a fidelity approach. In this situation, a combination of preordinate evaluation design and flexible data collection methods is required.

Thus an implementation evaluation may focus on factors affecting implementation—that is, the identification of conditions that encourage successful action. A motive for such a study could be to suggest ways of overcoming barriers to the implementation of the intervention.

Realistic evaluation

Realistic Evaluation is based on two fundamental propositions. The first is that evaluation studies should adopt a realist epistemology, which means that findings about the impact of a program are *generated* through inquiry. These findings take into account the context in which the program is implemented, and describe the processes or mechanisms that are responsible for the outcomes.

The second proposition is that it is not possible to ascribe universal or generalizable cause-and-effect statements about social programs. It is only possible to say that a program works under certain conditions. Paraphrasing this, a program is effective in certain circumstances for certain groups of participants in certain contexts.

These propositions follow from the view of Realists about the nature of change. They view program implementation as a complex process that will succeed only in so far as it introduces meaningful ideas and opportunities to groups in the appropriate social and cultural conditions. An implication is that implementation cannot be guaranteed; rather, it is providers and participants who must cooperate and make choices to make programs work.

Pawson and Tilley (1998) are among the chief advocates of the Realistic Approach. They reject the use of experimental methods to determine program impact, holding that use ignores the complexity of the intervention. Experimental methods do not allow for site-to-site implementation and differential take-up of participants in single sites.

The Realistic Approach includes the following stages:

1 The intervention needs to be clarified and examined. This involves evaluators identifying the logic of the program, using techniques outlined in Chapter 10.
2 Program (or policy) staff must be consulted early in the evaluation, rather than evaluators working from stated program intentions, or assuming that the program works as planned. This is to confirm the program logic that has previously been developed, and to create tentative hypotheses about how the program might affect the actions of providers and participants. These hypotheses are referred to by Pawson and Tilley as context-mechanism-outcome configurations.
3 Data management techniques that are sensitive to local site conditions and variations in implementation are employed. Pawson and Tilley are supporters of multiple methods and provide examples that include the use of exploratory case studies, sample surveys and 'realist experiments'.
4 Findings (or theory) consistent with the notion of 'what works for whom in a set of given circumstances' is developed from the findings. These are described as a 'specification', rather than a 'generalization' (Pawson & Tilley 1997, p. 86).

Realistic evaluation has been seen as a radical and important methodological design, but, there are critics who believe that Pawson and Tilley adopt an applied research rather than an evaluation perspective.

This is because of minimal involvement of stakeholders in the negotiation and utilization stages. However, we see no barrier to the incorporation of designs based on Realist principles into an evaluation framework.

Performance audit

The term 'audit' is well known to those familiar with the need for company accounts to be checked by a qualified accountant. The notion of auditing is associated with a review of financial arrangements—that is, a retrospective examination for the purpose of forming an opinion of their fairness in conformity with generally accepted accounting principles.

The term is now used more widely, signifying the adoption of auditing notions within other professions. We note the emergence of auditing methods that are not based on financial compliance—for example, an 'operational audit' is designed to provide management with an objective appraisal and opinions of all the activities of an organization, and may include recommendations for action.

Auditing procedures have also been used to examine the research output of government and university departments. For example, the administration of a large university commissioned external auditors to check all the research work undertaken by staff as a means of ensuring that the research met quality standards set by university funding bodies.

The Australian Universities Quality Agency (AUQA) has been established to assure the quality of tertiary education provision through independent audits. These examples lead us to the notion of performance auditing (PA), more generally defined as:

> a custom crafted analysis of program efficiency and effectiveness. It differs from financial auditing in that it deals with a combination of financial and non-financial measures and usually must define a unique set of measurements and standards for each audit that is undertaken (Brown et al. 1982).

According to Davis (1990), PA involves the:

> determination of the economy, efficiency, and effectiveness of government organizations, programs, activities and functions, in addition to their compliance with laws and regulations.

PA has also been defined as:

> an objective systematic examination of evidence . . . of the performance of a government organization, program or activity or function in order to provide information to improve public accountability and facilitate decision-making (Wisler 1996).

Evaluation theorists have become interested in comparing the work of program evaluators and auditors. Chelimsky (1985) contrasted the history and development of auditing and evaluation and compared methodologies used by practitioners in the two fields, and there have been subsequent contributions (see, for example, Davis 1990; Brooks 1996; Leeuw 1996).

There has been keen interest in the methods used in PA compared with those used in the objectives-based Approach (see, for example, Pollitt & Summa 1996). We must also review the epistemological basis of PA in order to locate it within the Forms framework. The practice of PA has been analyzed by Schwandt and Halpern (1998) as follows:

- a systematic process—an auditor's review and examination is planned, orderly and methodical;
- objectively obtaining and evaluating evidence—an audit is an independent empirical investigation;
- ascertaining the degree of correspondence between assertions and established criteria—auditing involves the exercise of professional judgment in applying a set of criteria;
- communicating the result to interested users—the outcomes of an audit examination is made public.

Based on a review of current practice, we see PA within the public sector being characterized by:

- considerable power to undertake an evaluation without the permission of agency or program managers;
- a strong emphasis on verification: the major role is to provide independent findings for accountability purposes;
- a focus on compliance and 'management' variables, plans and procedures;
- a focus on organizations as a whole, or on macro programs;
- a corresponding tendency to downplay the individual influence of components within an organization;
- an emphasis on reporting to outsiders: the primary audience is well defined and outside the program—for example, the legislature or parliament.

Comparing these developments with Approaches outlined earlier in this chapter, there seem to be sufficient similarities to acknowledge that PA is an evaluative Approach that fits within the Impact Form. PA should not only be embraced by those associated with the accounting profession, but also by those engaged in investigations in the helping professions when it is appropriate. For example, performance auditing has been used to review the curriculum in school systems in the United States (English 1988) and Australia (Owen et al. 1996).

In the public sector, there has been an increase in the proportion of effort spent on performance audits, compared with financial audits. Government auditors-general are seen as 'public watchdogs', reporting without fear to the legislature about the effective use of public resources. While their role as independent agencies has largely gone unchallenged, there are some politicians who believe that, in adopting the more evaluative roles associated with PA, auditors-general have exceeded their responsibilities.

This reminds us that evaluation work must take account of the political environment. Evaluation should be seen as important to any democratic society in that it should inform public policy, benefit those who make decisions about that policy, and inform citizens who have to live with those decisions, once made. Evaluators must make objective findings available, especially in a hostile political environment, and also when relevant public groups are unaware of the facts. It is up to evaluators because they have the ability to assemble the evidence and possess a commitment to the value of knowledge in decision-making.

Chelimsky (1995) believes that improvements and changes should be made according to whatever has been proven to be good, practical, desirable and meaningful, without an assumption that evaluators understand everything about the world and also know how to change it for the better. This is consistent with the Emergent Realist paradigm regarded as a philosophical basis for the conduct of evaluation, which was discussed in Chapter 5.

However, we would be naive to assume that all stakeholders in any political environment are likely to be open-minded, or willing to change their value positions, or share power, except in extraordinary circumstances. Rather, the norm is that political actors rarely put aside their agendas, and so evaluators need to work with those agendas, concentrating on securing the one thing that is most important for any evaluation in *any* political environment. This is the independence necessary to conduct their evaluations and state their conclusions without political interference (Chelimsky 1995).

Professional evaluators, including performance auditors, must deal with the fact that what we report in one political environment could be seen later on from the viewpoint of another. It is true that when policy is made in one environment, neither the policy nor the evidence evaluators bring to support it is likely to be without blemish. Policy and evidence cannot be perfect; instead, they are iterative and should be correctable. Rather than being seen as without fault, those involved in evaluation should be serious, credible and persistent. For those working squarely in the political arena, the challenge is to understand the strengths and vulnerabilities of both politics and evaluation and to use both of them to help us contribute to public policy in a meaningful and enduring way (Weiss 1999).

IMPACT EVALUATION: TRENDS AND CASE EXAMPLES

Determining outcomes in economic terms: Benefit for cost analysis

For some audiences, there is appeal in using simple measures to determine program worth. This resonates with those who subscribe to the view that a program should be judged in terms of its economic benefits. This effectively reduces the objectives of a program to a measure of efficiency: the more efficient the program, the more worthy it is. To employ methods consistent with this perspective, outcomes must be reduced to financial units of measurement.

Key notions associated with studies with this orientation include:

- benefit to cost ratio (BCR), defined as the ratio of program benefits to program costs;
- return on investment (ROI), defined as the ratio of net program benefits to program costs.

One area in which evaluators have encouraged greater attention to benefit to cost analysis is that of training in business and industry (Brinkerhoff 1989). In business terms, an imperative is to prove that training has contributed to the 'bottom line'. The following example adopted this perspective.

Example 13.1 A benefit for costs analysis of training

Phillips (1994) undertook an evaluation of a training program in a bank with offices across central states of the United States. The bank had a well-established loans section, which was in an expansion stage.

A training seminar on consumer lending for existing and new officers had been established within the Human Resources Department (HRD). The consumer lending seminar occupied three days. In the past, the HRD staff had always used reaction sheets for evaluation. However, senior management wished to see this program in terms of its benefit to the organization. The trainer and the manager of the HRD decided to take up the challenge of undertaking a benefit for cost analysis. A return on investment study was undertaken to meet this requirement. This involved making estimates of the costs and benefits in dollar terms.

- Program costs were as follows:

Instructors' and coordinators' salaries	$1,570
Admin. support	$500
Facilities, food, refreshments	$1,800
Participants' salaries (n = 20)	$7,200
Development costs (pro rata)	$300
Training materials	$400
Travel, lodgings, meals, etc.	$5,250
Other costs	$490
Total cost of seminar	$17,510

To calculate the impact of training, the evaluators:

- determined changes in the work effectiveness of the loans officers;
- allowed for changes by factors other than training which also affected the change in results.

Changes in effectiveness were obtained by collecting data on the 'before' and 'after' performance of each loans officer for a period of one year following the training. Where the officers were new, their performance in their previous job was traced. Where the officer had not been employed this way before, the average level of performance across the organization was assigned.

Factors other than training which influenced the effectiveness of the officers were reduction in interest rates during the year, and natural improvement—that which would have been likely to have occurred without the training. Corrections for these factors were made on the basis of data obtained from the bank. The key finding was that the loans officers finalized an increase of six loans per month after training, corrected for the above factors.

From the bank's records, it was possible to assemble the following information:

Average loan yield	9.75 percent
Average cost of funds	5.50 percent
Direct costs for consumer lending	0.82 percent
Corporate overhead	1.61 percent
Net profit per loan	1.82 percent
Average loan size	$15,500
Average monthly increase in loans per participant (corrected for other factors)	6
Number of participants in training seminar	18
Total amount of increased loans ($15,500 x 6 x 18)	$1,674,000
Annual improvement in loan values (x 12)	$20,088,000

Profit from improvement (x 1.82 percent)
$20,088,000 x .0182
$365,601
Return on investment (ROI)
= net benefits/costs
(365,601 – 17,510)/17,510
19.88

This is almost a 2,000 percent return on the training investment! Not surprisingly, this was regarded as extremely high by the HRD and the senior management of the bank, and ensured that the training seminar remained an integral part of the work of the Human Relations Department.

Treatment and control groups: Using variations in program provision to determine program worth

While some clients are content with outcomes in terms of cost benefits, others want more detailed information about the effects of a program.

One way to determine program effect is to invoke the use of an evaluation design based on the *experimental paradigm*. Borrowing from science, this involves the random assignment of subjects to two groups. One group undertakes the program (or treatment), while the other group, the control group, is not subjected to the treatment. By comparing the outcomes of the two groups, it is possible to reach a conclusion about the impact of the program. These are known as *laboratory studies* because, ideally, the implementation of the program is tightly controlled. Studies using this design also rely on the availability of a population of subjects from which the treatment and control groups can be drawn.

It is sometimes possible to find situations outside the laboratory where such principles can be used to evaluate a program. These are naturally occurring situations that approximate to an experiment, as defined above.

Example 13.2 Evaluating alternative modes of learning college physics

A college physics department became dissatisfied with courses provided for potential teachers. Several members of the staff became convinced that a 'traditional' course was no longer appropriate; what was required of science teacher preparation courses was a shift in basic philosophy and approach. A revised course was outlined which gave attention not only to physics knowledge and skills, but also—by its content, structure and presentation—to the nature of science in its social and historical context, and to the professional orientation of physics teachers. It was decided that a pilot version of the new course should be offered to an 'experimental' group of students, whose response and achievement would be compared with a control group taking the traditional course. Key evaluation questions were:

- Will the time given to the additional aims interfere to an intolerable extent with the students' acquisition of basic knowledge and skills?
- Can the new course be presented well enough that students perceive and develop towards the new goals?
- Will the students value the new approach in relation to their own perceptions of their personal and career futures?

The course presented to the control group was aimed at an understanding of the basic laws and theories of physics, an appreciation of their explanatory power, and skill in their application to solving physics problems. The course structure emphasized the logical structure of physics and was spiced with demonstrations and examples to help achieve these aims.

The course presented to the experimental group had three strands which ran side by side: one, the knowledge and skills of physics; another, discussions about physics; and the third, personal development and professional orientation through discussions about teaching physics.

Even though the two courses differed markedly in approach, their 'basic physics' aspects were similar in coverage and level of treatment. In this sense, the new course was an evolutionary development from the old, with many of the existing resources and ideas adapted to suit the new approach.

The evaluators compared the previous achievement in the areas of math and physics and found that the groups were similar.

After the courses were taught, it was found that the experimental group did no worse on achievement than the control group, despite the fact that they spent less time on basic concepts.

Both groups were also tested on another set of scales which measured laboratory skills, the ability to link physics with real-world problems, and a test of 'personal' skills, such as persistence in study. It was found that the experimental group performed considerably better on the first two of these additional tests.

The findings of this study were a key factor in having the new course adopted for all students (Hirst et al. 1980).

The need to establish actual program objectives

Sometimes when an evaluator is asked to undertake an objectives-based evaluation in the field, the objectives are not explicit. They then have to be determined by the evaluator before investigations of outcomes can be pursued. This is not an uncommon situation, for often developers do not provide well-developed objectives in program documentation.

Example 13.3 Evaluation of a Community Agency Human Development Program

For several years, the Richmond Community Health Centre (RCHC) has offered a unique program devoted to the discussion of issues such as contraception and the impact of drugs, aimed mainly at students in Year 11 (15–16-year-olds). Instruction was carried out by nurses and gynecologists at RCHC. The material covered and resources used in the program are not normally included in school curricula.

When the management of the RCHC found funds for an evaluation, the program providers (two nurses and a doctor) set the direction for the study. A major topic in initial provider–evaluator discussions was the potential use of the information from the study. It became clear that the providers had an agenda to produce information which could be used in negotiations at the RCHC and with funding agents to expand the influence of their program.

On this basis, it was considered essential to include a strong outcomes component and to spend less evaluation energy on an examination of program processes. In this case, the key outcomes issue was to determine whether the program was having an impact on students in terms of their knowledge and skills related to pre-pregnancy.

While there was extensive documentation on the program, there was no clear statement of objectives. To develop this, the evaluators interviewed the providers about their intentions and attended two program sessions. A member of staff no longer working on the program was asked to check trial items for their consistency with the intentions of the program. Thus the development of the final instrument relied more on interviews than on formal documentation of program objectives.

The need to convince outsiders of program worth led the evaluators to recommend the use of a simple pre-post achievement test design and the collection of testimonials from students and teachers involved. The fact that there was time for evaluation planning in advance of program delivery enabled careful matching of data management to the list of issues raised by the providers.

It was agreed that the providers would administer a simple instrument to students before and after each program session to measure achievement and to collect student opinions about the sessions. Further, it was decided that the evaluators would analyze these data, collect additional information about demand for the program over recent years from RCHC records, and design and carry out interviews with teachers responsible for the classes which attended the RCHC.

Data-collecting instruments were designed by the evaluators, who also undertook analysis for all phases of the study. The data collection methods and results included:

- an analysis of demand for the program over several years. This showed that more schools came from outside the educational region in which the Centre was located than from within it, and that up to 15 percent were country schools;

- the development and administration of a validated test of content covered by the program, included here as Figure 13.1. This was administered immediately before and then directly after the one-day course.

Figure 13.1 Richmond community program content test

Your ID Number ☐☐☐

RICHMOND COMMUNITY HEALTH CENTRE
PROGRAM REVIEW
Form Two

First, write your ID number, given to you on Form One, in the box above.

In this second questionnaire we would like you to answer the 'true/false' questions again and to give us some information about how the session was conducted. This will help us to make decisions about how good the course is and how to improve it.

Again, please answer every question even if you are uncertain or don't know.

1. A baby's estimated date of birth depends on the date of ovulation.

☐ True
☐ False
☐ Don't know

2. The major period of growth of the fetus (baby) is during the first months of pregnancy.

☐ True
☐ False
☐ Don't know

3. Most fetal organs develop in the first two months after conception.

☐ True
☐ False
☐ Don't know

4. The only signs of pregnancy are a missed period and morning sickness.

☐ True
☐ False
☐ Don't know

5. A baby's heart doesn't start to beat until at least 3 months into pregnancy.

☐ True
☐ False
☐ Don't know

6. Most problems in the formation of a baby occur either at conception or in the next few weeks.

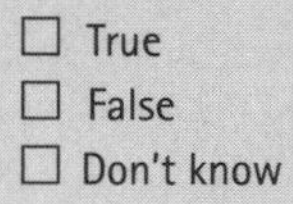

7. A woman need not be concerned about drinking alcohol or taking other drugs until she finds out that she is pregnant.

☐ True
☐ False
☐ Don't know

8. Most problems in the formation of a baby are caused by cigarette smoking.

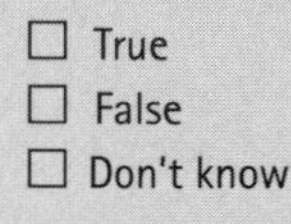

9. The only function of the placenta is to channel nourishment from the mother to the baby.

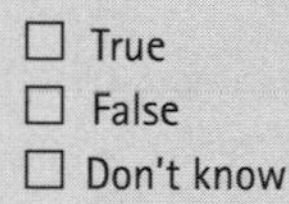

10. A baby has little chance of survival if born before the 22nd week of pregnancy.

☐ True
☐ False
☐ Don't know

11. Babies can be born small and undernourished if the mother smokes heavily during pregnancy.

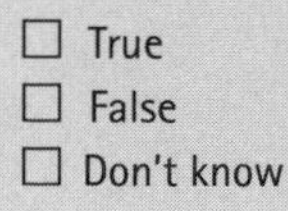

12. Babies can be born deaf or blind if the mother suffers from rubella (German measles) in early pregnancy.

☐ True
☐ False
☐ Don't know

13. Babies of drug addicts suffer withdrawal symptoms after birth.

☐ True
☐ False
☐ Don't know

Now, we would value *your* opinions of the session.

14. What is the most important thing you have learnt from today's session?

____
____
____
____

15. What was the best aspect of the session? Why?

(You might like to think about the content, presentation, or the organization of the morning.)

____
____
____
____

16. What was the worst aspect of the session? Why?

(You might like to think about the content, presentation, or the organization of the morning.)

____
____
____
____

17. Have you any comments to make about the video(s) you saw? Please write them below.

____
____
____
____

18. If you wish, please suggest one way in which the session could have been improved. (You might like to think about the content, presentation, or the organization of the morning.)

____

____

____

____

Before you hand this second questionnaire in be sure that you have written your ID number on the top of this questionnaire and that you have answered every question.

The results showed that:

- the average gain scores of the participants was statistically significant;
- increased scores occurred for students from all schools;
- almost equal gains were made by male and female students;
- there were variations in gains between items on the test, which suggested that some sections of the course had been more successful than others;
- some items were answered well on the pre-test which indicated that they need not be included in any future course.

Opinions about the program were sought from students and their teachers, focusing on the 'best' and 'worst' aspects of the program. The most frequent student response in the first category was an appreciation of the style of presentation. Students liked the friendly, informal atmosphere of the classes and straightforward manner with which issues were dealt.

A follow-up interview with all participating teachers found that information about the program most frequently came from other teachers, that the program was used to complement and reinforce what was being done at school, and that the visit was treated as an adjunct to subjects taken at Year 11 level in areas such as Home Economics, Human Development and Society, and Human Studies.

Besides presenting these results, the evaluation also made recommendations relating to the development of more appropriate videotape support material, the criticisms being that the imported tapes used were not entirely appropriate for Australian audiences, and that they were factually incorrect and out of date (Hurworth et al. 1988). This issue emerged early in the teacher interview phase, and its exploration required follow-up by cross-checking with health center staff.

In this case, the findings were used to argue a case for the introduction of this course in other health centers. The evaluators agreed to join providers in presentations of findings to various health agencies. The extent of evaluator commitment to this phase was determined by the strength of the findings. If the impact of the program had been small or negative, the evaluators may not have adopted a strong dissemination role.

This example highlights an evaluation in which the implied goals of a program formed the basis for a major aspect of the evaluation. It is evident from the description that additional evidence was collected in order to provide comprehensive information for decision-making. It is also notable that data were collected in a variety of ways and in different formats.

Surrogate measures of outcomes

As indicated earlier, a standard procedure in outcomes-based evaluation is to develop outcomes measures that have strong face validity. However, there are situations where compromise is required. This involves the use of surrogate measures, which substitute, or stand in place of, preferred or ideal measures. If one uses such surrogate measures, an argument must be made in terms of their validity when presenting the evaluation findings. This was the case in Example 13.4, in which an outcome indicator was used as a surrogate for direct learning to evaluate the impact of a health education program.

Example 13.4 Evaluation of the impact of a health education program for ethnic mothers

Among staff at Inner City Health Center, there was concern about the quality of nourishment provided within local non-English-speaking households. After extensive consultation with these families, the center implemented a program aimed specifically at women with small children from an ethnic group. The program, offered in two-hour evening sessions, was intended to:

- promote a return to eating traditional food of the ethnic group;
- promote breast-feeding (all participants had at least one child under two years of age);
- reduce the extent of obesity among children in the families.

Over the eight weeks of the program, the ten participants were given information, through an interpreter, designed to change existing approaches to feeding their children.

A short time after the program had been completed, the Health Center decided to commission a small-scale evaluation of the impact of the intervention.

Assisting providers to identify key evaluation issues was a prerequisite to detailed evaluation design. The major audience was the administration of the Center. In this case, a genuine need emerged to discover whether this pilot program had led to a change in the nutrition intake. In identifying this issue, the evaluators recommended the collection of simple indicators of impact.

However, there were problems in choosing and collecting the most appropriate data caused by the limited resources for the study and its timing vis-à-vis program delivery; in this case, the evaluation was *post hoc*.

One suggestion was to follow up the participants using an interview or a questionnaire. There were difficulties envisaged in using either of these approaches. These included negotiating access to the women within the context of traditional ethnic households, problems of translation, and finally—even if these difficulties were overcome—issues relating to accurate and open recall of information about the program.

Doubts about the reliability of the data collected by these means led the evaluators to consider alternative data sources. The evaluators became aware that it is an almost universal for mothers to take their babies the Health Center for periodic check-ups.

Documentation included a running record of infant physical development, including weight charts. Given that a major aim of the program was to reduce the obesity of children in the families, the evaluators decided to use changes in weight of children as indicators of the impact of the program. The Health Center was assured of confidentiality in the use of these records.

The availability of the charts allowed the evaluators to follow two lines of investigation.

The first involved variations in weight of the ten young children born before the program began. The analysis charted variations from birth through the period of the program, and subsequently during the ten months following its conclusion. Inspection of the charts, included as Figure 13.2, showed that the weight of children in these families was consistently above the median before the program, that it fell during its duration and then maintained a trend close to the median after program conclusion.

On the basis of this analysis, the evaluators were prepared to conclude that the program had been a success, at least on the grounds of reducing obesity among the children.

However, it was felt that further information should be collected to be more certain of the conclusion that the program had a lasting impact. Through discussion with program staff it was found that three of the families had produced an additional child subsequent to the program. As before, charts were investigated and showed that the weights of these children followed the median from birth. We were thus more certain that the program had left a lasting impact on these families.

The evaluators prepared a 'user-friendly' report and ensured that all members of the Health Center became aware of the findings through seminars and discussion. Despite the problems inherent in the *post hoc* nature of the evaluation, the findings were seen by the audience as strong grounds for the Center staff to be confident that their program had a lasting impact on the participants. Subsequent to the findings of the study becoming known, the evaluators encouraged the Health Center to apply for funding to conduct the program again. This application was successful and the program ran again the following year (Hick 1988).

This case illustrates the need for evaluators to solve difficult methodological and ethical issues. Some commentators say that a good evaluation has a touch of artistry and creativity, and this could be regarded as a case in point.

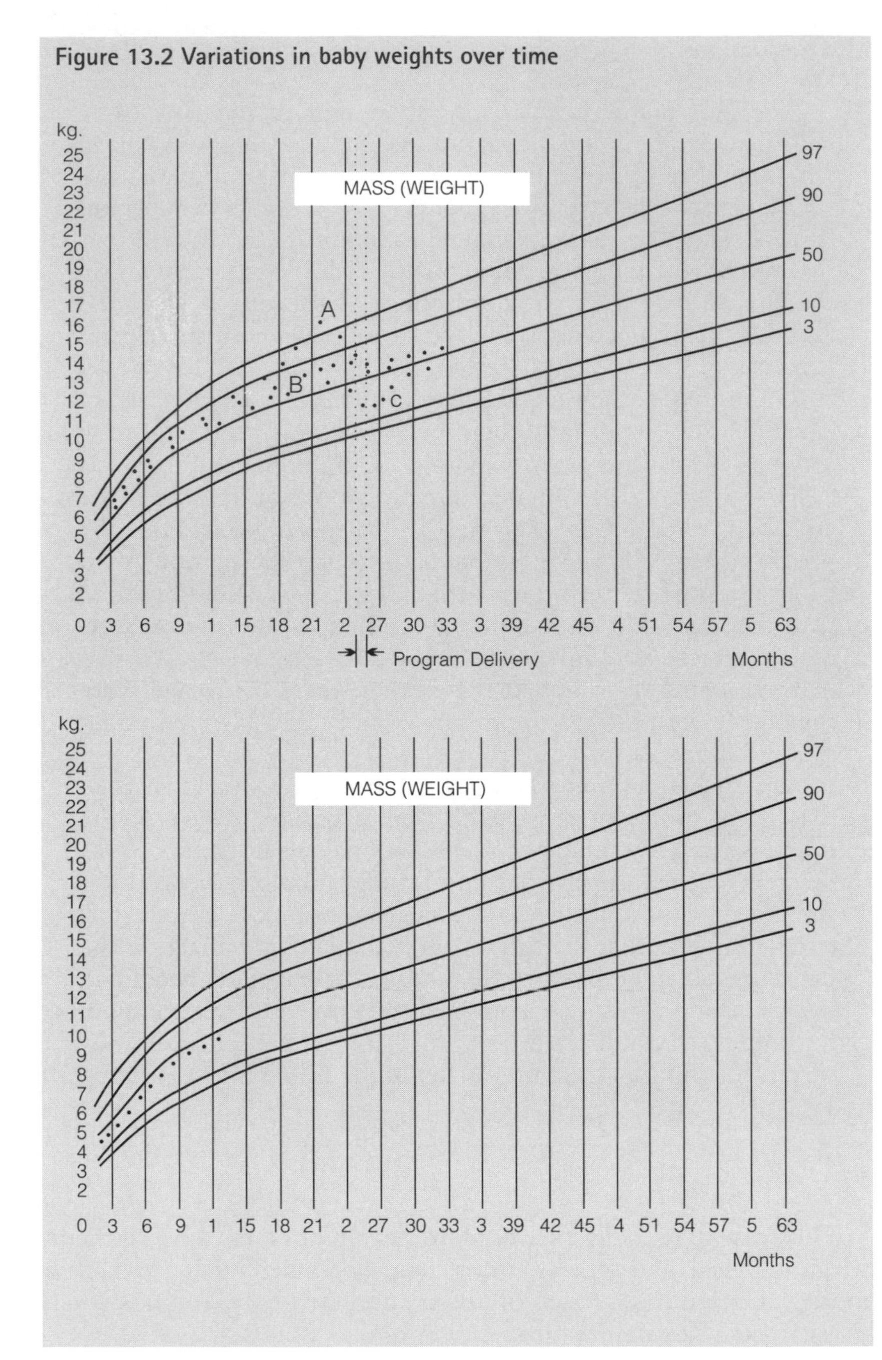
Figure 13.2 Variations in baby weights over time
kg.
MASS (WEIGHT)
A
B
C
97
90
50
10
3
0 3 6 9 1 15 18 21 2 27 30 33 3 39 42 45 4 51 54 57 5 63
Program Delivery
Months
kg.
MASS (WEIGHT)
97
90
50
10
3
0 3 6 9 1 15 18 21 2 27 30 33 3 39 42 45 4 51 54 57 5 63
Months

Needs-based impact: Finding a suitable external criterion for judgment

As indicated earlier, needs-based Impact evaluations are rare. This is due in part to the fact that few needs assessments are actually carried out in advance of program planning and development. It is also true that many program developers base their planning decisions on other factors besides empirical findings, relying more on their 'local knowledge', or the way they prefer to deliver their programs, or on an ideological view of acceptable practice. These issues provide a challenge for an evaluator to establish a framework from which an assessment of impact can be made on the basis of need, as illustrated by Example 13.5.

Example 13.5 An evaluation of alternative courses within a teacher education program

A large college offered five alternative courses within a one-year teacher education program. The extent of variation in the program was based on an argument that there was no 'best way' to educate a prospective teacher. However, dwindling resources and other factors led the college to a view that the range of choice and diversity was no longer acceptable. An evaluation was undertaken to inform course committee debate about which courses should remain and which might be discontinued.

The key issue which underpinned the evaluation was to determine the relative effectiveness of the courses in preparing students for their first years as schoolteachers. It was therefore necessary to develop outcome measures of effectiveness, and to develop ways of determining the effectiveness of the alternative courses in preparing students to be effective beginning teachers. These issues were a focus of discussion within the college.

There was a concern to develop procedures for fairly judging the relative worth of the alternative courses, not on their own terms (that is, relative to their objectives), but on grounds which allowed the courses to be compared.

The issue was solved satisfactorily by reference to a recently completed national inquiry into teacher education. The inquiry recommended a core of learning experiences that should be required of all students and was effectively a policy statement to guide teacher education. The availability of these guidelines provided a set of common criteria for making comparisons between courses. The course committee endorsed this approach and decided that beginning teachers should be a major source of information, given that they had participated in one of the courses and most of them were now working in schools.

A survey, included as Figure 13.3, was sent to all graduates eight months after they had completed the program.

Figure 13.3 Diploma in Education course evaluation

1. What team did you belong to in the Diploma in Education course at the College? (Check one)

☐ A	☐ B	☐ C	☐ D	☐ E	☐ F
(part-time)	(core-elective)	(school-based)	(contract-based)	(elective-based)	(community-based)

2. Please list your method studies

____________________, ____________________, ____________________

3. Which of the following activities applies to you in 1983? (Check one or more)

☐ Teaching full-time ☐ Teaching part-time ☐ Student ☐ Other job ☐ Unemployed

If you are teaching (full- or part-time) go to QUESTION 5 and complete the remainder of the checklist.

4. *IF YOU ARE NOT TEACHING AT ALL* please state briefly the reason why you are not teaching this year (be as specific as possible).

THIS COMPLETES THE CHECKLIST FOR THOSE NOT TEACHING THIS YEAR.
THANK YOU FOR YOUR ASSISTANCE.

5. Listed below is a series of items which describes aspects of teaching. On the left-hand side indicate the emphasis each was given during your teacher education year. On the right-hand side we would like you to evaluate each aspect according to its current *importance to you in your present position (as a teacher).*
PLEASE RESPOND TO EVERY QUESTION.

Emphasis in my teacher education year (Check one)		↓	*Importance to my present position (Check one)*
Little/None	☐	i) An ability to control classes which I teach	☐ Not Important
Small	☐		☐ Slightly Important
Moderate	☐		☐ Moderately Important
High	☐		☐ Very Important

Emphasis in my teacher education year (Check one)			*Importance to my present position (Check one)*
Little/None	☐	ii) An ability to translate a curriculum plan into action	☐ Not Important
Small	☐		☐ Slightly Important
Moderate	☐		☐ Moderately Important
High	☐		☐ Very Important
Little/None	☐	iii) An ability to evaluate my own teaching performance	☐ Not Important
Small	☐		☐ Slightly Important
Moderate	☐		☐ Moderately Important
High	☐		☐ Very Important
Little/None	☐	iv) An ability to plan a curriculum unit which I will teach	☐ Not Important
Small	☐		☐ Slightly Important
Moderate	☐		☐ Moderately Important
High	☐		☐ Very Important
Little/None	☐	v) An awareness of the ways schools can develop closer relations with the community	☐ Not Important
Small	☐		☐ Slightly Important
Moderate	☐		☐ Moderately Important
High	☐		☐ Very Important
Little/None	☐	vi) A knowledge of factors affecting the intellectual development of adolescents	☐ Not Important
Small	☐		☐ Slightly Important
Moderate	☐		☐ Moderately Important
High	☐		☐ Very Important
Little/None	☐	vii) Insights into the interconnections between subjects offered in the school curriculum	☐ Not Important
Small	☐		☐ Slightly Important
Moderate	☐		☐ Moderately Important
High	☐		☐ Very Important
Little/None	☐	viii) Sensitivity to the range of disadvantages students might face in schools (on the bases of ethnicity, gender, socio-economic background or physical handicap)	☐ Not Important
Small	☐		☐ Slightly Important
Moderate	☐		☐ Moderately Important
High	☐		☐ Very Important
Little/None	☐	ix) A knowledge of factors affecting the emotional and social development of adolescents	☐ Not Important
Small	☐		☐ Slightly Important
Moderate	☐		☐ Moderately Important
High	☐		☐ Very Important
Little/None	☐	x) A knowledge of recent developments in 'method' areas related to my subject specializations	☐ Not Important
Small	☐		☐ Slightly Important
Moderate	☐		☐ Moderately Important
High	☐		☐ Very Important

Emphasis in my teacher education year (Check one)			*Importance to my present position (Check one)*
Little/None Small Moderate High	☐ ☐ ☐ ☐	xi) An ability to cater for the strengths and weaknesses of individual students	☐ Not Important ☐ Slightly Important ☐ Moderately Important ☐ Very Important
Little/None Small Moderate High	☐ ☐ ☐ ☐	xii) An awareness of the relationship between schools and the broader social/political context	☐ Not Important ☐ Slightly Important ☐ Moderately Important ☐ Very Important
Little/None Small Moderate High	☐ ☐ ☐ ☐	xiii) An ability to work with students in different settings (classroom, excursions, camps etc.)	☐ Not Important ☐ Slightly Important ☐ Moderately Important ☐ Very Important
Little/None Small Moderate High	☐ ☐ ☐ ☐	xiv) An understanding of the organization and structure of education in Victoria	☐ Not Important ☐ Slightly Important ☐ Moderately Important ☐ Very Important

6. Now, please use the space provided below to make any comments on your *teacher education year*, in the light of your subsequent experiences. *Please be as specific as possible.*

i) Strengths:

____

____

____

____

ii) Weaknesses:

____

____

____

____

iii) What changes would you recommend to the teacher education year you undertook?

____

____

____

____

7. Finally, could you tell us how satisfied you are with your present teaching position?

☐ Very satisfied ☐ Moderately satisfied ☐ Slightly satisfied ☐ Not at all satisfied

Write a note to explain your response if you wish:

____

____

Information was sought about, first, the degree to which core learning experiences were covered in the course they undertook at college; and, second, the degree to which each of these were perceived as important to them as beginning teachers. Fourteen items were written to cover the core learning experiences. From the replies (N = 165, 80 percent response after telephone follow-up), it was possible to determine the discrepancy between importance and emphasis for all items on the survey and the relative degree to which the program as a whole emphasized

Figure 13.4a Evaluation of college teacher education program

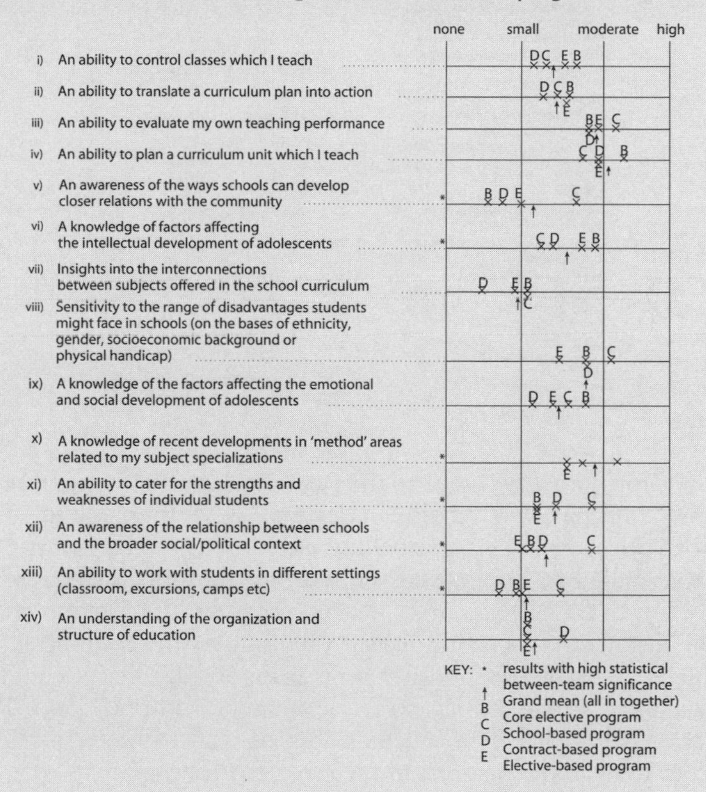

each core learning experience, as indicated in Figure 13.4a. This information enabled comparisons to be made between items, and allowed high discrepancies between importance and emphasis to be identified. Figure 13.4b compares the emphasis of each course on all items. Open-ended responses supported the statistical information that showed Course C was the most effective in preparing teachers for the workplace.

Figure 13.4b Evaluation of college teacher education program—emphasis

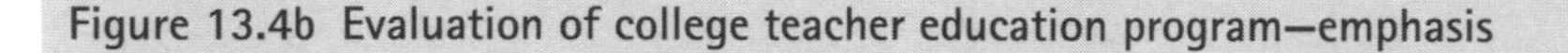

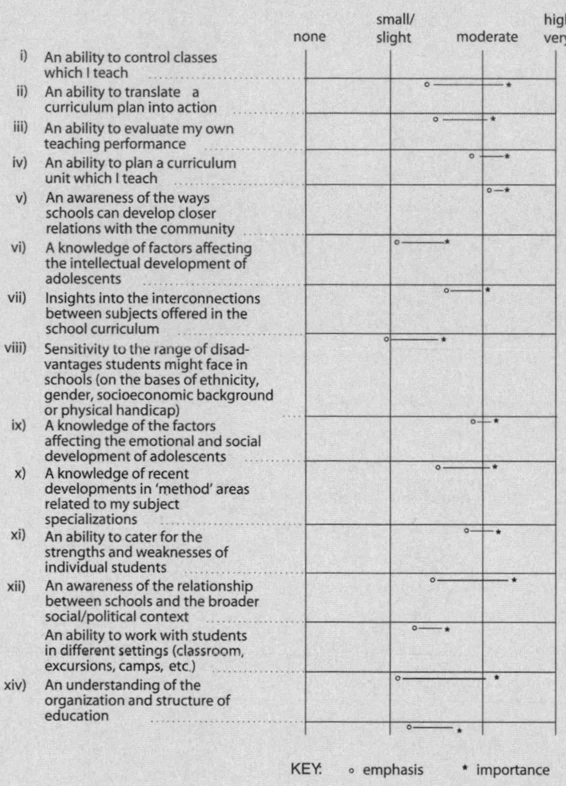

A short paper was sent to the Program Course Committee in which findings, *not* recommendations, were highlighted. The information provided compelling reasons to retain Course C, the so-called 'school-based' course which was judged to be superior to the other courses, within the program. The information became the focus for decision-making by the committee, in which one of the evaluation team was involved. They effectively saved this course, which was about to be scrapped on other bases, such as it was too demanding of staff to be in the field rather than in the institution for most of the week.

The findings of this study made an immediate and identifiable difference on decision-making. Example 13.5 relied on a strategy of examining the effects of a program in terms of the way it prepared participants to function effectively in employment subsequent to its delivery. This is analogous to evaluating goods and services in terms of effective usefulness criteria, an approach used in consumer magazines.

The design is highly appealing as a basis for undertaking impact studies. The difficulty of translating these principles into action, however, is testified to by the paucity of needs-based impact studies in the literature.

Managing impact studies of 'Big P' Programs

Federal agencies responsible for the delivery of macro or 'Big P' Programs often have an evaluation component built in to the funding agreement. The size and breadth of a 'Big P' Program provides a challenge for evaluators if they are asked to undertake an Impact study. This is due to factors such as:

- Big P Programs are often delivered at many sites, at different locations often widely spread across geographical areas;
- individual site-level programs can also be delivered at different times; and
- the intentions of an individual 'small p' program offered within the umbrella of the 'Big P' Program may not reflect the objectives of the umbrella program.

There is also the problem of encouraging local staff to cooperate with the large-scale evaluation effort. The study described in Example 13.6 managed to surmount these problems. By developing generic outcomes, and using a range of person-intensive procedures, a quality database was developed from which across-site findings were assembled.

Example 13.6 Evaluation of training programs of the Center for Substance Abuse Prevention

The Center for Substance Abuse Prevention (CSAP) leads a major effort in the United States to prevent substance abuse, which has been linked to concerns about increased community violence, rising need for health care, teenage pregnancy and decreased work productivity. CSAP administers a range of programs by contract. Training is a key program on the CSAP agenda.

Due to the interest in the impact of training, a large-scale five-year longitudinal study of the CSAP Training System (CTS) was undertaken by Ottoson (1994) and her colleagues. CTS training focuses on building the capacity of individuals and community organizations to plan and carry out prevention programs. During 1994 and 1995, about 9,500 participants participated in CTS training across America. Training ranged in length from half a day to five days. The evaluation represented a major effort to tap the opinions and intentions of all participants in almost 250 separate interventions. The findings of the study enabled decision-makers to judge the effect of each program and, by aggregation, the total training Program. In addition to evidence collected immediately after training, 2,100 respondents were followed up two months after training was completed. Generally, respondents reported positive reactions immediately post-training. On a ten-point scale, used to indicate the extent to which participants were disposed to apply learning from the sessions, the mean score was 7.7. The follow-up data showed that the respondents were engaged in a broad range of selected prevention activities. A feature of the reporting was the classification of open-ended responses into seven categories of intervention. These were: learning; information dissemination; education; providing healthy alternatives; problem identification and referral; involvement in community-based processes; and influencing the environment. These categories had been developed by the parent agency of CSAP, the Substance Abuse and Mental Health Services Administration (SAMHSA) (Ottoson 1994).

This study has a similarity to that outlined in Example 13.5, in that a set of 'generic' outcomes was developed as the basis for data collection that enabled aggregation and comparison across 'little p' programs. In this case, outcome criteria were drawn from common expected features of all programs and from the literature on effective training.

Process–outcome studies

Reports of process–outcome studies are hard to locate, because few evaluations using this Approach are carried out, and even fewer are reported in evaluation journals. As indicated earlier in this chapter, studies require assessment of implementation and outcomes and, if possible, evidence which shows those aspects of implementation that lead to the outcomes. We have noted that implementation is a complex and time-consuming task, almost always involving the evaluator in intensive observation of program delivery. This means that impact studies involving implementation usually involve a small number of sites unless there is a large team of observers available. Having only a small number of sites also affects the way we make an inference about cause and effect. If there were a large number of sites, we could use a between-site correlation to determine the size of the link. If we have a small number of sites or indeed just one, we must rely on analyses that do not rely on statistical inference. Example 13.7 illustrates such a situation.

Example 13.7 Implementing Roadsmart

Roadsmart is an educational package designed to improve the safety of road behavior of students.

This program consisted of approximately twelve hours of in-class teaching to students, tuition outside which included practice in road crossing, and the education of parents on major issues of road safety. Two teachers were trained to deliver the program. An evaluation involved intensive recording of the road-crossing behavior of all students in the two classes before the program began, using hidden video recorders. Data were then collected two weeks after the program had been completed.

In addition, the evaluator spent time at the school watching the delivery of the program and the teachers kept notes on how they taught each session. Outcome evaluation focused on student behavior.

The evaluator found that students adopted far more effective crossing behavior after the program, watching more closely and spending less time on crossing. It was found that both teachers implemented most of the activities suggested by the program designers; however, one teacher spent much less time on most of the activities. There was no difference in the behavior of the students in the two classes, which suggested that the quality of student experience was more important than the length of time taken to complete the program. Justification of the link between implementation was made with recourse to the fact that changed behavior of the students was unlikely to have been due to any environmental effect in the period in which the program was taught (Leadbetter 1998).

It should be noted that Example 13.7 employed a preordinate design. The approach to studying implementation was based on the intentions of the program, which formed the basis of the observation schedule used by the evaluator. In Example 13.8, the evaluation, while noting program intentions, used a less structured methodology to determine program impact.

Example 13.8 Evaluation of the Frontline Management Initiative (FMI)

The Frontline Management Initiative (FMI) was designed to assist staff with middle-level management responsibilities to improve their skills in conjunction with carrying out their day-to-day tasks.

A state department of the environment trialed the FMI in twelve regional sites across the country to assist decision-making about adopting the Program more widely. An independent evaluation was commissioned in which the evaluators:

- developed a program logic from documentation available;
- interviewed key stakeholders, and in particular human resource personnel, to obtain a sense of how the FMI was functioning;
- monitored the take-up of the FMI over a period of about a year. Evidence was collected through site visits, interviews and document analysis. Extensive use of matrices enabled large amounts of data to be collated and analyzed.
- found large between-site differences in implementation, which were explained by factors such as: site-level support of local management, matching between the FMI and pre-existing site-based needs, and the effectiveness of the training team that was commissioned to work at the site.

This example reflects principles of the Realist Approach described earlier in this chapter, in that context, processes (or mechanisms) and outcomes were able to be linked at both site and individual levels (Owen et al. 2001). In this case the evaluators also assisted stakeholders to consolidate the integration of FMI into the management processes of the department.

There is sometimes a naivety about implementation among funding agency staff and senior management, who believe that, once resources have been allocated to a given social intervention policy, the program can be assumed to be in place. A not-uncommon scenario is one in which senior management, often under political pressure, expects program staff to plan and implement a program within extreme time constraints. The reality is that working through an idea or policy to develop implementation guidelines is often complex. The consequent step of translating guidelines into action then requires support and time to ensure that the program makes an impact in the field. Without these steps, incomplete or partial implementation is a real possibility.

In summary, implementation studies should occupy a strong place in evaluation practice, because we need to find out what is actually taking place during program delivery. This applies whether or not the program is disseminated from a central agency or is developed locally.

CONCLUSION

The conclusion of a final chapter of a treatise is an appropriate location to look back over what has been presented, in this case to reflect on the evaluation concepts and examples of practice presented. The reader should now appreciate that the notion of evaluation which grounds these concepts and examples represents an extension and broadening of meaning compared with those presented by other evaluation theorists. The resulting paradigm summarized by the Evaluation Forms is largely a response to criticisms that conventional evaluation theory and practice has not fulfilled the expected promise in achieving social betterment (Schwandt 2002).

The rationale adopted here is unashamedly utilization focused and on the production of knowledge that is relevant to program decision-making. This is illustrated by the focus on working with clients and understanding their agendas, and thus, the attention given to planning, negotiation, and dissemination strategies. It is true that these elements have been emphasized by other evaluation theorists, but they have been largely confined to those who subscribe to a participatory paradigm. It is our view that these elements need to be present in work done within (and across) all Evaluation Forms. This sometimes requires evaluators to insist on procedures that may not have been expected by commissioners of evaluation studies. Evaluators must then play an educative role as a basis for convincing commissioners and other program stakeholders about the benefits of negotiation as a trade-off for the resources required to ensure that the evaluation agenda is clear before the evaluation design is implemented. While some might question the ability to maintain the critical independence required to present accurate findings, our experiences over a period of almost two decades of practice is that the vast majority of clients will respect evaluators conclusions developed under these conditions, even if they contain unpleasant messages for program stakeholders.

Finally, it is worth re-asserting the reality that evaluation findings are usually one input into program and organizational decision-making. While it is clear that we value the contribution of empirical inquiry highly, we also recognize the important contributions that other types of knowledge must play in organizational milieux. It is the judicious combination of evaluative findings with professional expertise and grounded experience that makes for effective decision-making, organizational improvement, and social betterment.

REFERENCES

Auditor-General, Victoria. (2004). *Beyond the Triple Bottom Line: Measuring and Reporting on Sustainability*. Melbourne: Victorian Auditor-General's Office.

Brinkerhoff, R. (1989). Evaluating training in business and industry. *New Directions for Program Evaluation*, 44, 5–19.

Brooks, R. A. (1996). Blending two cultures: State legislative auditing and evaluation. *New Directions for Program Evaluation*, 71, 15–28.

Brown, R. E., Gallagher, T. P. and Williams, M. C. (1982). *Auditing Performance in Government*. New York: John Wiley.

Chelimsky, E. (1985). Comparing and contrasting auditing and evaluation: Some notes on their relationship. *Evaluation Review*, 9(4), 483–503.

Chelimsky, E. (1995). The political environment and what it means for the development of the field. *Evaluation Practice*, 16(3), 215–25.

Davis, D. F. (1990). Do you want a performance audit or a program evaluation? *Public Administration Review*, 50(1), 35–41.

English, F. W. (1988). *Curriculum Auditing*. Educational Resources Information Center (ERIC) Microfiche ED 302 912.

Guskey, T. R. (1994). Results-oriented professional development: In search of an optimal mix of effective practices. *Journal of Staff Development*, 15(4), 42–50.

Hall, G. E. and Loucks, S. F. (1979). *Innovation Configuration: Analyzing the Adaptations of Innovations*. Austin, TX: Research and Development Center for Teacher Education.

Hick, P. (1988). 'An evaluation of a nutrition program for young Turkish mothers.' Unpublished paper for the Graduate Diploma in Adult and Continuing Education, Melbourne College of Advanced Education.

Hirst, R., Malcolm, C. and Owen, J. M. (1980). An example of evaluation in the development of a tertiary physics program. *Research in Science Education*, 10, 151–7.

Hurworth, R. E., Owen, J. M. and Griffin, L.D. (1988). *The Impact of the Richmond Community Health Centre Pre-Pregnancy Program*. Melbourne: Centre for Program Evaluation, The University of Melbourne.

Leadbetter, C. (1998). Roadsmart—an evaluation. Unpublished Master of Education Thesis, The University of Melbourne.

Leeuw, F. L. (1996). Auditing and evaluation: Bridging a gap, worlds to meet? *New Directions for Program Evaluation*, 71, 51–60.

Morris, L. L. and Fitzgibbon, C. T. (1978). *How to Measure Program Implementation*. Beverly Hills, CA: Sage.

Ottoson, J. (1994). *Training Evaluation Report of 1994 Profile, Feedback and Follow-up Data*. Vancouver, BC: prepared for The Training and Evaluation Branch, Division of Community Prevention and Abuse Prevention, Center for Substance Abuse Prevention.

Owen, J. M., Meyer, H. and Livingston, J. (1996). *School Responses to the Curriculum and Standards Framework*. Carlton, Vic: Victorian Board of Studies.

Owen, J. M., Meyer, H. and Lazenby, K. (2001). *The Natural Resources and Environment Experience of FMI: An Evaluation*. Melbourne: Centre for Program Evaluation.

Pawson, R. and Tilley, N. (1997). An Introduction to scientific realist evaluation. In E. Chelimsky and W. Shadish (eds), *Evaluation for the 21st Century*. Thousand Oaks, CA: Sage, 405–418.

Pawson, R. and Tilley, N. (1998). *Realistic Evaluation*. London: Sage.

Phillips, J. J. (ed.) (1994). *In Action: Measuring Return on Investment*. Alexandria, VA: American Society for Training and Development.

Pollitt, C. and Summa, H. (1996). Performance audit and evaluation: Similar tools, different relationships? *New Directions for Program Evaluation*, 71, 29–50.

Rugg, D., Peersman, G. and Carael, M. (2004). Editors' notes. *Global Advances in HIV/AIDs Monitoring and Evaluation*, 103, 1–11.

Schwandt, T. A. and Halpern, E. S. (1988). *Linking Auditing and Meta-evaluation*. Beverly Hills, CA: Sage.

Schwandt, T. A. (2002). *Evaluation Practice Reconsidered*. New York: Peter Laing Publishing.

Scriven, M. (1972). Goal-free evaluation. In E. R. House (ed.), *School Evaluation: The Politics and the Process*. Berkeley, CA: McCutchan.

Spillane, J. P., Reisner, B. J. and Reimer, T. (2002). Policy implementation and cognition: Reframing and refocusing implementation research. *Review of Educational Research*, 72(3), 387–431.

Tyler, R. (1950). *Basic Principles of Curriculum and Instruction: Syllabus for Education 360*. Chicago, IL: University of Chicago Press.
Weiss, C. H. (1999). The interface between evaluation and public policy. *Evaluation*, 5(4), 468–486.
Wisler, C. (1996). Evaluation and auditing: Prospects for convergence. *New Directions for Program Evaluation*, 71, 1–5.

INDEX